SCARS

SCARS

WHAT DRS. DIDN'T TELL THEM

REAL PATIENT STORIES

LINDA DUNN-CARTER LE, CPCP

White Falcon Publishing

SCARS
Linda Dunn-Carter LE, CPCP

Published by White Falcon Publishing
Chandigarh, India

First Edition, 2024

Cover design by White Falcon Publishing, 2024
Cover image source Linda Dunn-Carter LE, CPCP

ISBN - 979-8-89222-225-9

CONTENTS

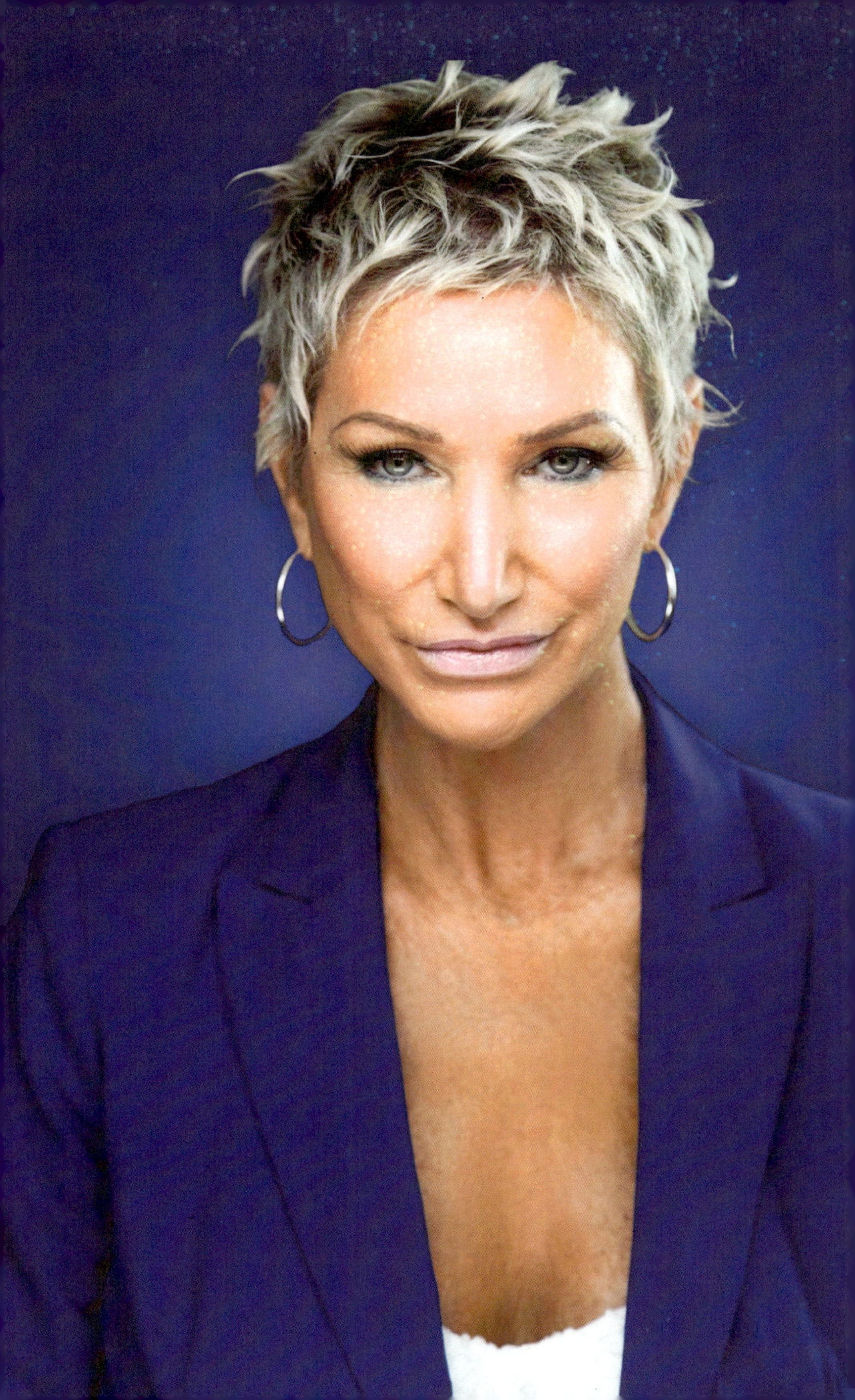

PREFACE

My name is Linda Dunn-Carter, LE, CPCP, and I have made it my life's mission to treat people with scars.

The DC Method was created in 2006, and since then, I've performed over 65,000 procedures using my own techniques designed to minimize or eliminate scarring. My new book, SCARS: WHAT **DRS. DIDN'T** TELL THEM, is designed to be a resource for anyone who is considering surgery or looking to have their old scars revised naturally. Photos (some graphic) are of my actual patients, and the information is based on my professional experience, case studies and patient results. My goal is to treat everyone in need, one scar at a time.

In this book, I'll tell you how your skin type can affect your risk of scar complications. I'll also share how to conduct your own critical research, how to prepare for the all-important consultation with your prospective surgeon, and lastly, share some crucial aftercare tips that are beneficial for all surgeries. My team and I can assist with pre-surgical and post-surgical treatment plans that most surgeons don't provide.

I would like to express gratitude to all my patients over the years who have helped me perfect and achieve results beyond my dreams. A special thanks to my courageous patients who have shared their intimate scar journeys in the SCAR STORIES written and featured in this book. I have printed their stories verbatim from their interviews, which I hope will help many readers understand that there is always hope for changing the appearance of their scars. I would also like to thank the surgeons, dermatologists, and peers who refer their patients and clients to me for expert care. Additionally, I am grateful to Dr. Marty Zaiac and Anne Gueta for their professional support during the peak phases of my career, as well as Plastic Surgeon Dr. Pamela Brownlee, Plastic and Reconstructive Surgeon, and trauma specialist, and J'Adore Mattis, MSN, APRN, FNP-DC, for contributing their wisdom on the importance of scar risk education and the need for better access to postoperative scar care.

CHAPTER 1
HOW DO YOU SCAR?

HOW WELL DO YOU KNOW YOUR BODY?

Unfortunately, in skin and scarring, we are not all created equal. Many of my patients often tell me, "If only I had known the risks, I never would have had the surgery!" The plain, unmitigated truth is that many surgeons don't volunteer the critical information their patients need.

That's why I'm calling this book SCARS: WHAT **DRS. DIDN'T** TELL THEM. Many of my scar patients were completely unprepared for the extent of their scar complications. Why are we not surprised? Because their doctors never informed them about the risks. I often see patients after the damage has already been done, and that damage can be devastating.

This book will empower anyone considering surgery by teaching them the basics and also where to go to find the information that will make them well-informed about surgical and scar repair choices. One of the first steps in an individual scar journey is to understand what type of skin you have and how prone your type of skin is to scarring.

Understanding your skin and your risks will help you ask intelligent questions before you have surgery or attempt to revise any pre-existing scars. You will begin to understand the importance of having a Scar Plan that identifies and treats your particular type of skin.

> **PRO TIP**: "Don't expect your surgeon to volunteer information about your scar risks; you must ask the question if it's not offered." – *Linda Dunn-Carter*

So, are you ready? Let's get started on your personal scar journey. I've prepared some examples of skin types that will help you identify your own skin type. These examples, along with my actual patient photos, will also help you visualize how different types of skin have significantly different scar risks.

Keep in mind that having proper scar care pre-op and post-surgery can mitigate the risk of some of the worst complications.

GETTING TO KNOW YOUR SKIN

Let's walk you through what you need to know. Skin types are categorized according to the Fitzpatrick Scale. You can find additional details about the Fitzpatrick Scale on Wikipedia. This scale takes into account the amount of pigment or coloration in your skin, as well as how your skin reacts to sun exposure. It also predicts the level of scar risk for each skin type. It's important to note that different skin types can react differently to various kinds of trauma, such as surgery or accidental injury.

PRO TIP: "People with darker skin tones, such as African Americans, Hispanics, Asians, and those of Mediterranean descent, have a higher risk of developing dark, thick scars. They are also more prone to forming keloids, where the scar grows outside its normal boundaries. It is especially important to discuss this with these patients before surgery and have a well-defined scar plan in place for post-surgery." – *Dr. Pamela Brownlee, Plastic and Reconstructive Surgeon*

CAN YOU RECOGNIZE YOUR SKIN?

On the Fitzpatrick Scale, there are two types of pigments or "Melanin" that combine to make up these skin types: Red-Brown for Fitzpatrick scale 1-2, and Brown-Black for Fitzpatrick Scale 3-6: All skin types are at risk of some kind of abnormal healing post-injury, but the risk factors multiply in darker skin. For example, scars in lighter skin can hyper or hypo-pigment, become atrophic, or turn red, while darker skin is more vulnerable to major scar complications such as hypertrophic scarring, keloids, and hyperpigmentation (see photos). If you have higher-risk skin, don't be discouraged because we are here to help with your newfound knowledge of risks and appropriate pre-op and post-op scar care. With these advantages, the risk of scar complications can be addressed with a high rate of success.

TYPE I

SKIN COLOR - White
HAIR - Blonde, Strawberry Blonde, Red
EYES - Green
SUN EXPOSED - Can't Tan, Always Burns, Freckles
SCARRING - There is a low risk of scarring. In the long term, healing is relatively good. Scars can either be flat and the same color as the surrounding skin, or flat and white, indented and white, or they may remain red for extended periods of time, depending on the depth of the injury. Raised scars are rare.

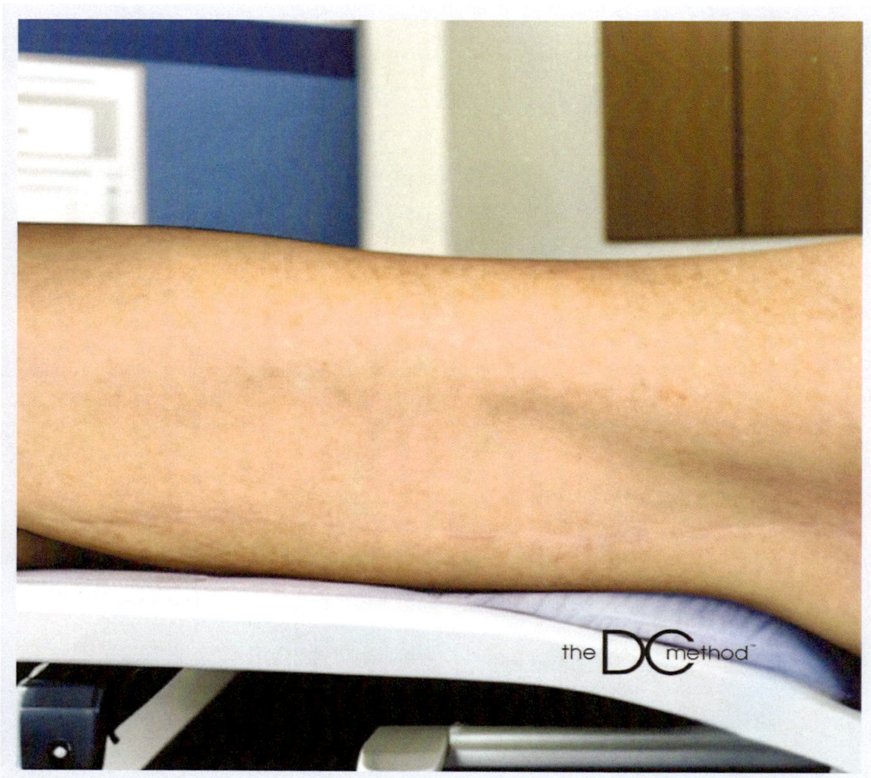

Skin Type I

TYPE 2

SKIN COLOR - White
HAIR - Blonde, Strawberry Blonde, Red
EYES - Green, Blue, Light Brown
SUN EXPOSED - Mostly Burns, Freckles, Difficult to tan.
SCARRING - Low to medium risk of scarring. Long-term healing is relatively good. Scars can be flat and the same color as the surrounding skin (which is rare), flat and white, indented, textured, or remain red for extended periods of time, depending on the depth of the injury. Raised scars are rare.

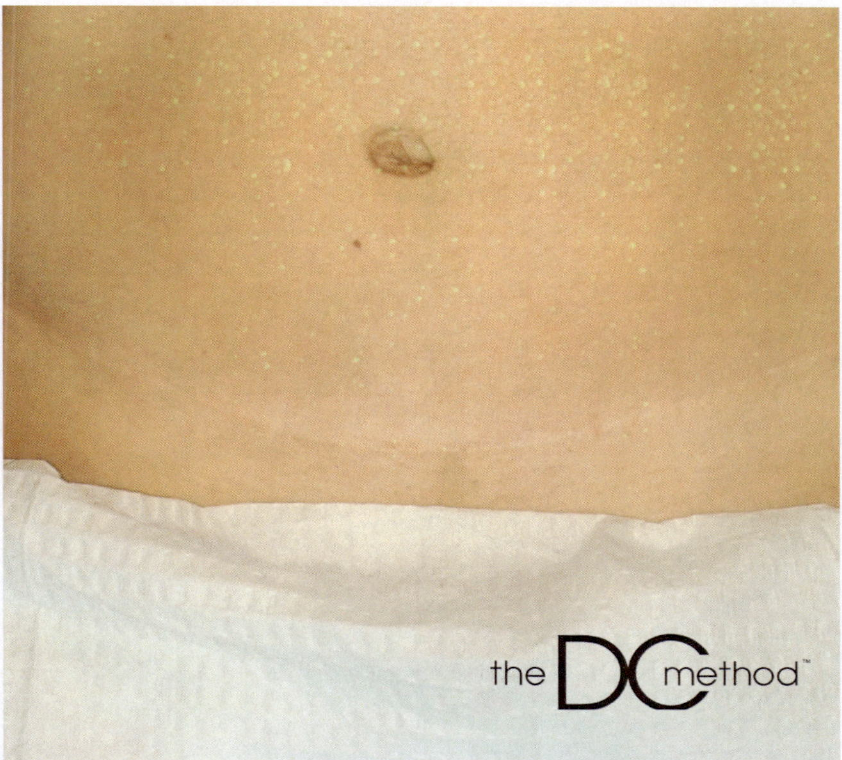

Skin Type 2

TYPE 3

SKIN COLOR - Slightly darker than Type 2 with golden undertones.
HAIR - Blonde-Light Brown
EYES - Green, Blue, Brown
SUN EXPOSED - Tans easily. Can burn when in the sun longer, but eventually turns to a tan.
SCARRING - Prone to an increase in melanocytes, which can result in a higher likelihood of scarring after an injury. Possible effects include raised scar margins, hyperpigmentation, hypopigmentation in the center or furrow of the scar, as well as flat and white, flat and dark, raised and dark, or uneven skin.

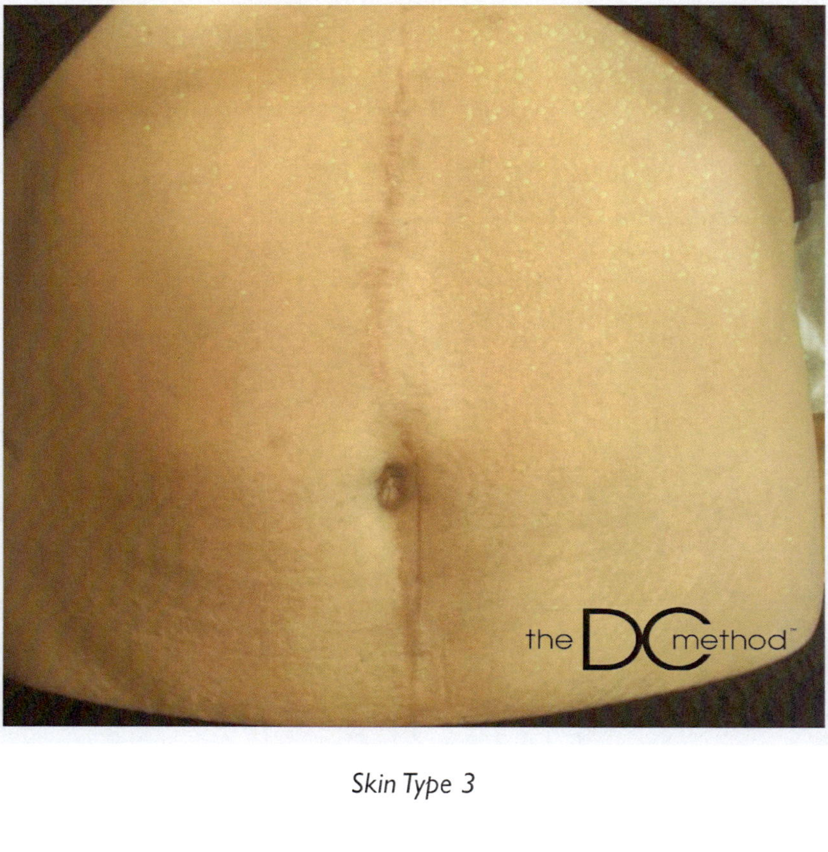

Skin Type 3

TYPE 4

SKIN COLOR - Olive or caramel. Browner.
HAIR - Brown
EYES - Brown or Hazel
SUN EXPOSED - Tans easily. Can still burn with prolonged exposure to the sun.
SCARRING - Scars easily. Scars can easily turn dark at the margins and migrate beyond the injury site or incision. They can be flat and white, flat and dark, raised and dark, or keloid.

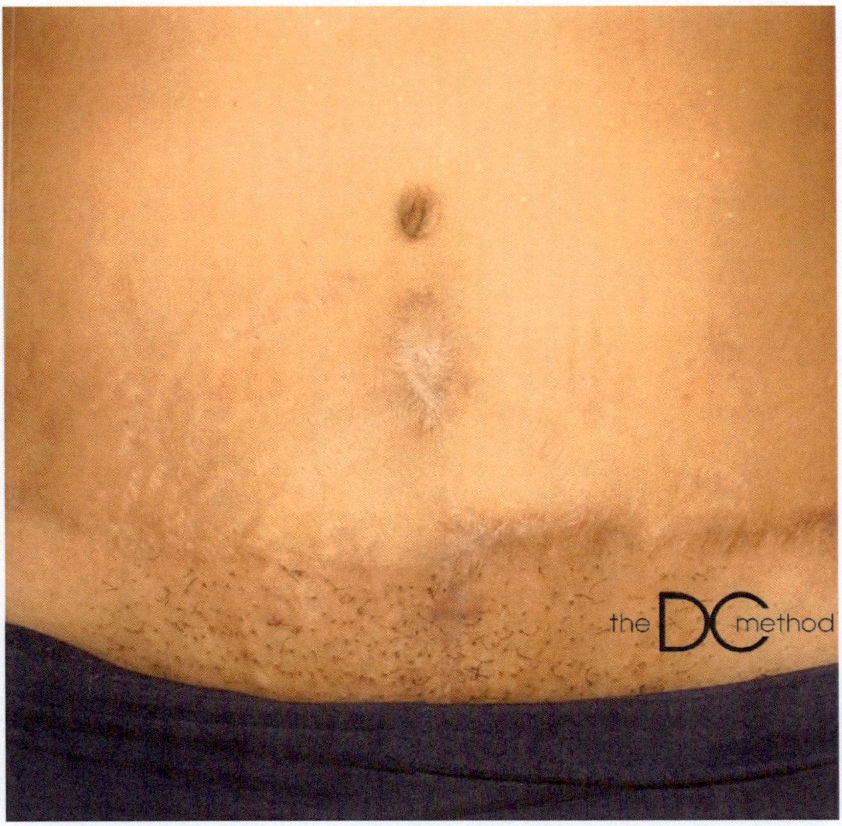

Skin Type 4

TYPE 5

SKIN COLOR - Dark Brown
HAIR - Brown or Black
EYES - Brown
SUN EXPOSED - Tans easily. Rarely burns.
SCARRING - Scars easily. Scars can easily form and may darken at the edges and extend beyond the original injury site or incision. Scars can appear flat and white, flat and dark, or a combination of both dark and white. They can also be raised and dark, or even keloid scars.

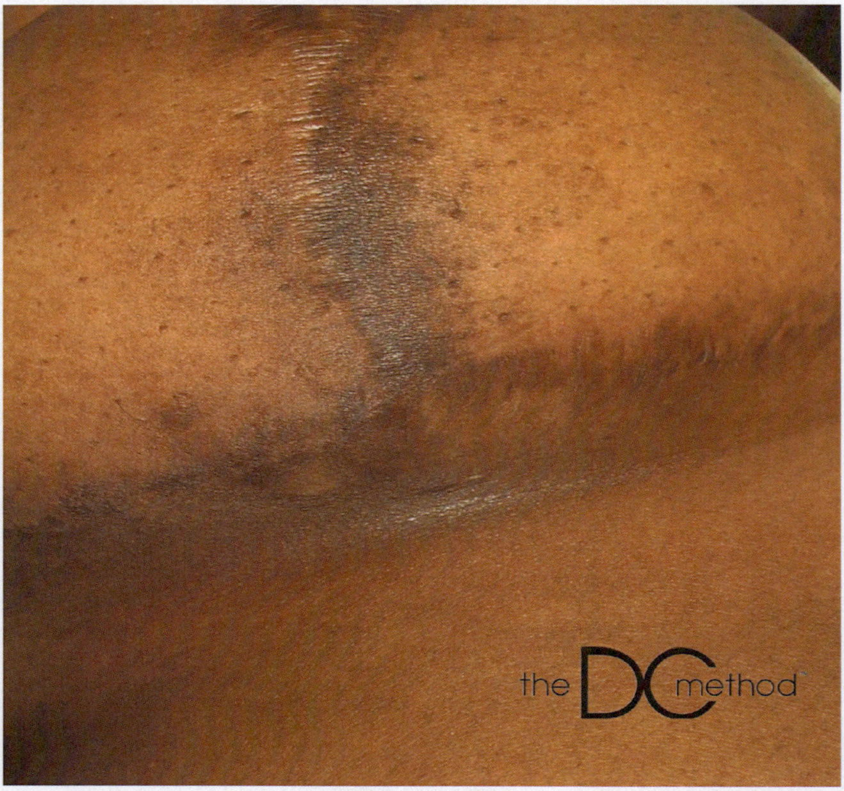

Skin Type 5

TYPE 6

SKIN COLOR - Mahogany or Black
HAIR - Black
EYES - Brown
SUN EXPOSED - Tans easily.
SCARRING - Scars are abnormal. Scars can become extremely dark at the margins, and the darkness can spread beyond the site of the injury or incision.
They can be flat and dark, raised and dark, or keloid. Rarely white.

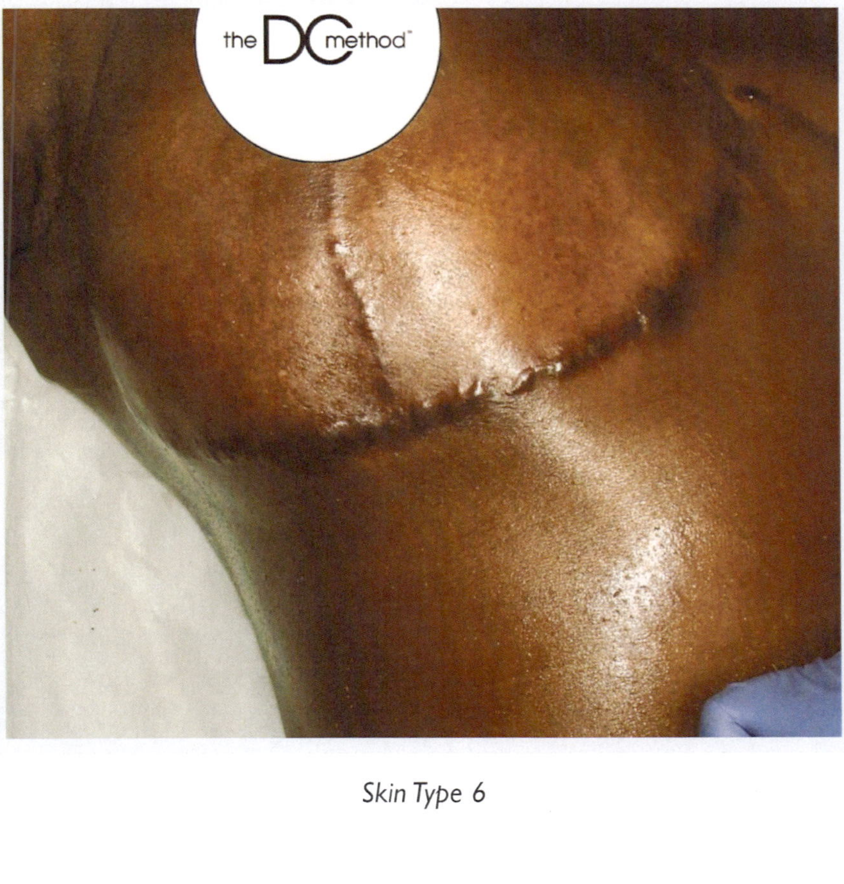

Skin Type 6

PRO TIP: "Surgery equals scarring. There's no such thing as scarless surgery." – *Linda Dunn-Carter*

So, as you are now abundantly aware, we are not all made the same. Frankly, less than 5% of the population will likely heal well without a scar intervention plan that considers skin type and overall risk. When the scalpel cuts through the skin or you injure yourself, there will be a scar. How you heal is based on factors such as your hereditary background, preventative care, aftercare, your general health, and often the quality of how your incision is sutured. Since it's clear that there's a lot your doctor won't tell you, according to my patient's stats, I feel it's important to cover many of the missing details in the coming chapters of this book.

WHAT ABOUT YOUR PERSONAL SCAR HISTORY?

If you know that you tend to heal poorly, this is valuable information that you should definitely discuss with your surgeon. Even if it's the smallest of injuries, like a keloid from a piercing or a hypertrophic scar from a childhood fall, there could be important clues about how you might heal after future surgery. Also, the size of the scar can multiply the extent of complications. An 18" tummy tuck scar can be challenging if not managed properly. The sides might heal fine, but the middle might experience extreme tension, causing the incision to open during healing and resulting in a much wider scar. The longer the incision, the more complications can arise. Additionally, keep in mind that how you heal on your face might not be how you heal on your lower body and extremities. There is more blood flow and gravity to the lower part of your body, which can cause more tension on your incision. Extra tension on healing skin can also lead to complications.

SCARS: WHAT DRS. DIDN'T TELL THEM. The quality of your surgeon's suturing has a major impact on how you heal. So, do you happen to know if your surgeon is planning on doing the suturing? Or will they assign this critical detail to a staff nurse or surgical assistant? Will they be readily available if complications do occur? Some of my patients have been asked to follow up remotely with a virtual Physician's Assistant, even after serious complications! Make sure your surgeon doesn't have a history of disappearing once the fee is paid and the surgery is done.

WEIGHING YOUR OPTIONS

Popular plastic surgery procedures, such as breast lifts, tummy tucks, and arm lifts, carry the risk of major scarring complications. It is advised to carefully weigh the pros and cons of potential surgical risks before making a commitment. Always take into account your personal medical history when considering these risks. For instance, if you have previously undergone surgery and are prone to spitting sutures, keloids, and hypertrophic scarring, it is likely that any new incision will present similar issues.

You need to weigh these risk factors and decide if you are prepared to take on the challenge if things go wrong.

PRO TIP: "If you have a high-risk scar profile, you always have the option to reconsider elective surgery." – *Linda Dunn-Carter*

SCARS: WHAT DRS. DIDN'T TELL THEM will provide readers with a detailed guide to critically important information in upcoming chapters. Meanwhile, all of my scar patients just assumed that there was no hope for their devastating surgical scars. The good news is that with a personalized scar plan and proper care, any scar can be on a healthier path to a better aesthetic appearance.

The DC Method™ provides patients with versatility and can address both old and new surgical scars. Reach out to our Hotline at 866-SCARTLK for a consultation, scar revision services, product information, or training. We're here to assist you. Every scar is important to us, and every question has an answer.

CHAPTER 2
THE EMOTIONAL TOLL

WHAT IS THE EMOTIONAL TOLL WHEN SCARS DON'T HEAL?

We all have them: minor scars from the falls we had as kids, acne scars, and more serious scars from things like accidents or surgery. Ninety-five percent of scars are permanent to some degree. Sure, some scars will simply fade, but less than five percent of people heal well enough that you won't notice their scars. This means that the majority of people live with some type of visible scarring after trauma or surgery. What many people do not realize before voluntarily choosing surgery is that the emotional and psychological impact of scar complications can be devastating and long-lived unless you have a scar plan.

HOW SEVERE ARE THE PSYCHOLOGICAL SCARS ON THE INSIDE?

According to a document from PubMed [pubmed.ncbi.nlm.nih.gov]: "Those with scars undergo remodeling of their emotional state and are more prone to the development of depression and anxiety;

feelings of shame and aggression can follow. This creates strain in social interactions, resulting in stunned communication, reduced intimacy, and avoidant behaviors."

PRO TIP: "A scar can hurt both physically and mentally. It can be a constant reminder of a traumatic event, whether it is from cancer, surgery, or an accident. Seeing the scar day after day can take a mental toll on someone, reminding them of a terrible time in their life." - *Dr. Pamela Brownlee, Plastic and Reconstructive Surgeon*

So, what are the options to relieve the physical, emotional, and psychological marks of scars? Fix them! In my mind, it was really that simple. My job is multifaceted as a scar revision expert: to manage new scars and repair old ones, and ultimately give my patients back their confidence and peace of mind!

Every scar has a story, and every story is just as important to me as the one before. You could say I'm part healer, part coach, part advocate, and most importantly, a scar expert.

When patients with scars following cosmetic surgery (tummy tucks, breast lifts, and burns) arrive at my clinic, they are often completely devastated by the appearance of their scars.

Many people have given up hope and are seriously depressed. Their scars have impacted their relationships and careers, shaking them to the core. I advise them that with a well-thought-out plan and patience, we will witness improvement. I have a multitude of before and after photos of similar scars to share with them, followed by the preparation of a comprehensive treatment plan.

THE PATH TO HEALING

With time, their confidence grows. I become very close to my patients during the long periods of time together as I'm healing their scars. As their scars change physically from the outside, it is clear that the physical and psychological transformations are undeniably linked. Progress on the outside can lead to renewed self-confidence and restore a patient's sense of self. As one of my patients commented, "I feel like me again!"

SCAR STORY #1 – CESIA'S INTERVIEW

Yeah, so I started this journey about ten years ago. I had implants on my breast. And then after several years, I got tired of them because they were too heavy. So in 2017, I saw a doctor (plastic surgeon). He is well known here in Miami for doing very good surgeries. I was very confident doing my surgery with him because he had this amazing reputation. So we did what is called an ex-plant (removing breast implants).

WHAT MY DOCTOR DIDN'T TELL ME. No one prepared me for complications. And after two months, three months, I started getting keloids on my scars. So honestly, I thought and I felt that I had to live with them for the rest of my life. I didn't know what it was, you know? I was ashamed to look at myself in the mirror. It was very shocking to live with these keloid scars for so long, from 2017 until 2022.

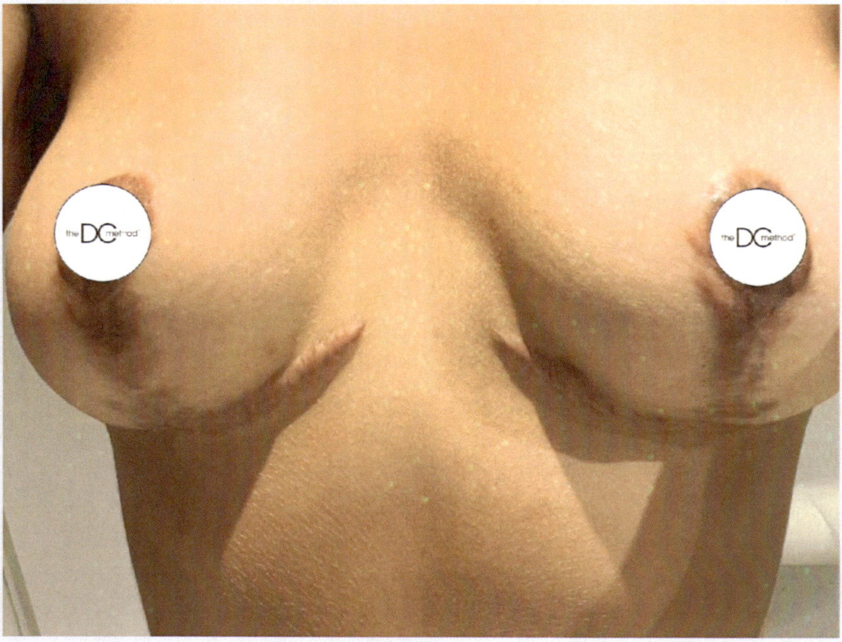

Cesia: Before Revision to Remove Keloids and Widespread Hypertrophic Scarring

Then in 2022, I was having dinner with a couple of friends of mine. And one girl, she started mentioning that she had keloids and that she went to see this woman who is amazing and that she treats keloid scars. And I was like, "Wait a second! That sounds like my story, you know?" I said to her, "Adriana, what is it that you're saying?" She says, "I had terrible keloids and Linda, she's amazing. She's here in Miami and she's been treating my scars." So I went to the bathroom with Adrianna. You know, I'm like, "Oh my God, I need to see this in person." So she showed me the before and after photos on her Instagram page. And I said, "Wow! I never thought that someone was going to be able to help me with my scars. I never thought that this was going to be possible, you know?"

She gave me Linda's number, and I sent an email. Linda then sent me a questionnaire of things that she needed to know prior to seeing me. Three weeks later, she finally saw me, and my scars were severe.

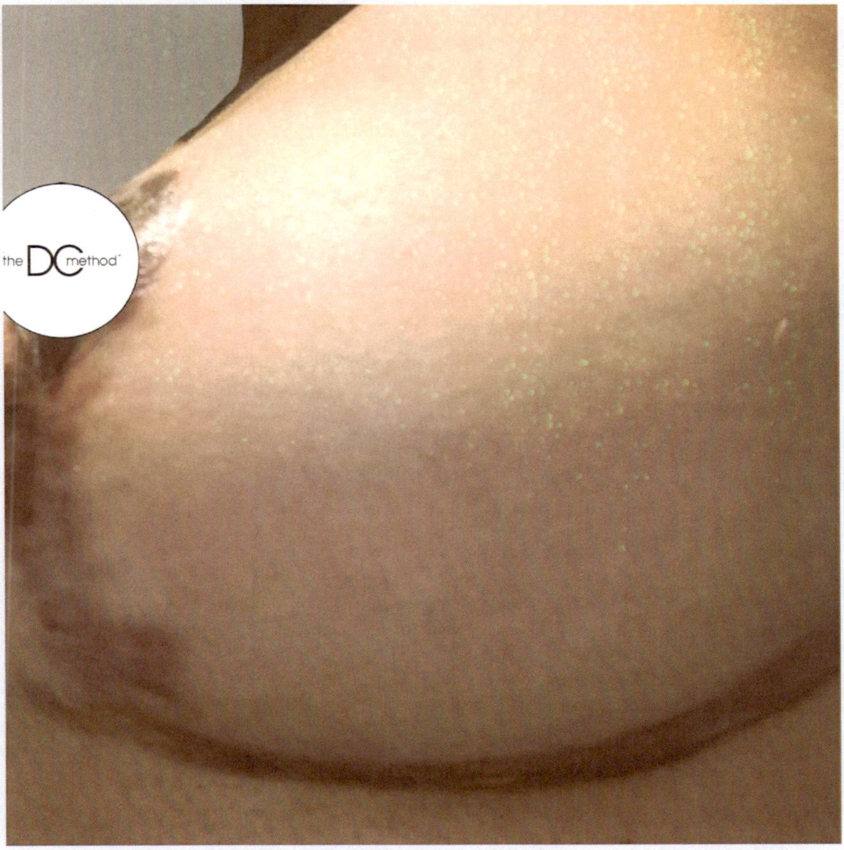

Cesia, Left Side Before Revision:
Severe Keloids and Widespread Hypertrophic Scarring

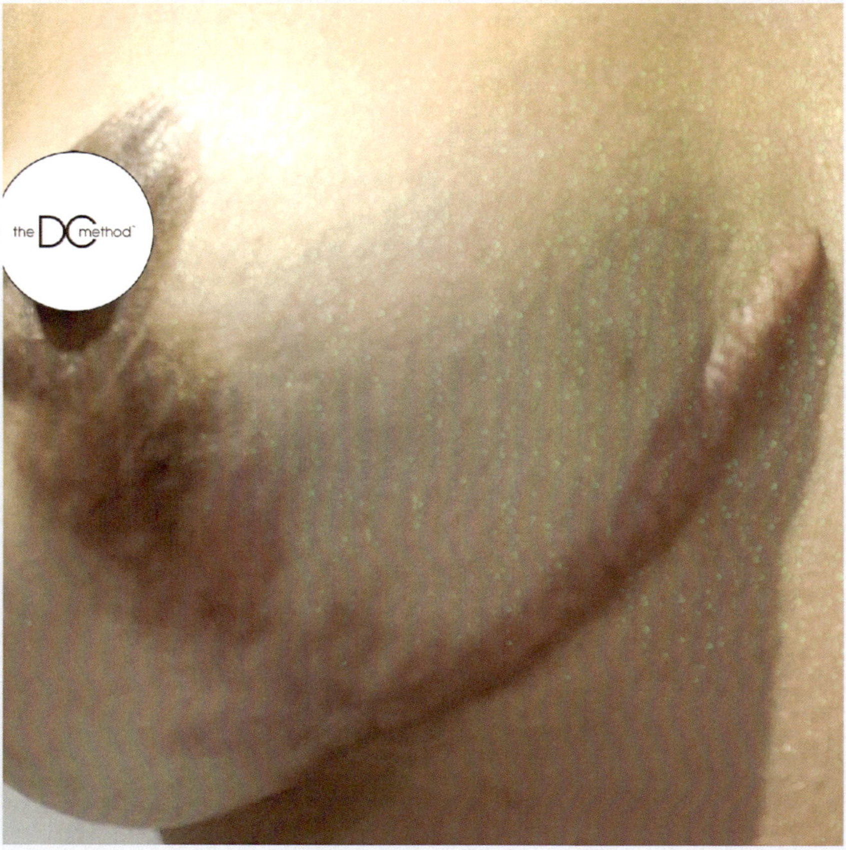

Cesia, Right Side Before Revision:
Severe Keloids and Widespread Hypertrophic Scarring

Since it was such a long time and since I didn't do anything about them, I had to go through another surgery. But this time, I had a plan with Linda. She said, "You're going to come see me two days after your surgery and we're going to do this,' you know, 'We're going to do several procedures after the big revision procedure," which was the surgery to treat the scars. And that's exactly what we've been doing for a year.

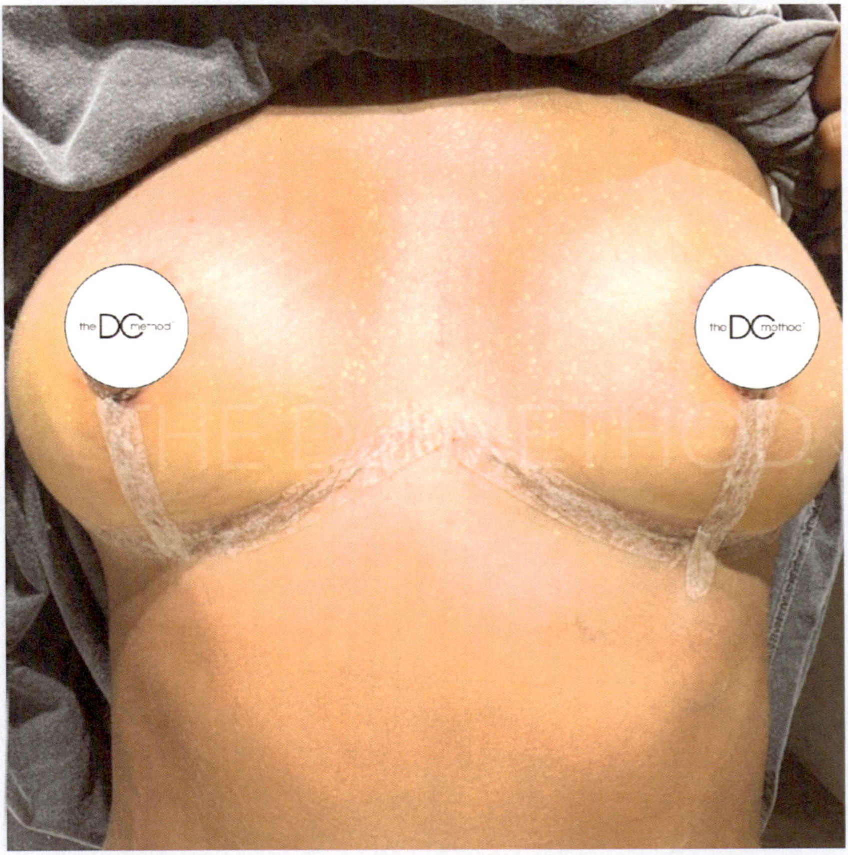

Cesia, Immediately After Revision Surgery

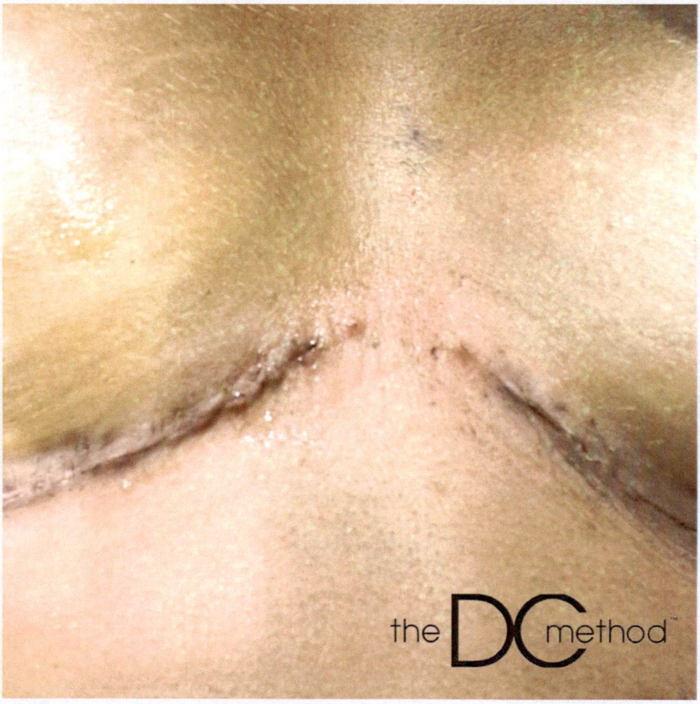

Cesia, After Tape Removal: Areas of Concern where her original keloids were removed

WHAT MY DOCTOR DIDN'T TELL ME. But this is the thing, and Linda and I talk about it all the time. People think that by going through another surgery, the scars will not come back and that is a total myth about these keloids. No, it doesn't work like that. You need to have a plan! You need to follow up, you need to do these treatments. That's exactly what we did.

The very next day I sent her pictures, and she could see raised areas through the wound tape which of course could very well be keloids trying to form. So guess what, she had to come back early to Miami. She's amazing like that. Like when she gets a patient.

She takes it very seriously. You know, I wish that the surgeons would pay attention to this, but they honestly don't care.

They only care about performing the surgery, and that's it. They don't care about the scars!

Linda said that since we were going to treat the scars, it didn't matter who did the surgery. So, I went back to him, the same surgeon. And when he saw me with the scars, he said, "Oh, who was your previous doctor?" And I said, "You did it; you were." And he said, "Oh, I did that?" Weeks after we had the surgery, they wanted me to come back, but I never wanted to talk to them again.

You just can't understand how bad it was to live like that with the keloids.

My sexual life was just destroyed. (Before) you know, I never felt very confident with my partner. And then those five years I just had to, you know, wear a bra, not allow him to see me... I couldn't even see myself naked in the mirror because I was traumatized. I just knew I needed to be with her (Linda): As long as I needed to get this over with, you know? She didn't mention how long the series would take and I didn't ask.

Linda: Cesia came to me with severely debilitating keloid scars. After five years in this terrible state, she had given up any hope of finding help until a friend referred her to me. Her self-esteem was at rock bottom, and she was even ashamed to show her naked body. I was confident I would get better aesthetic results, but I also knew it would require scar revision surgery. After the revision, new keloids started to form within days, but we were ready with a plan. It was more than a challenge to stay on top of the dozens of keloids that popped up after her revision, not to mention spitting sutures that festered underneath her skin. But now, more than 16 months later and managing all these issues, her new scars are 90 percent better than her original keloid scars. She is back to her proud, self-confident self, and I couldn't be happier for her. What a joy to have Cesia back!

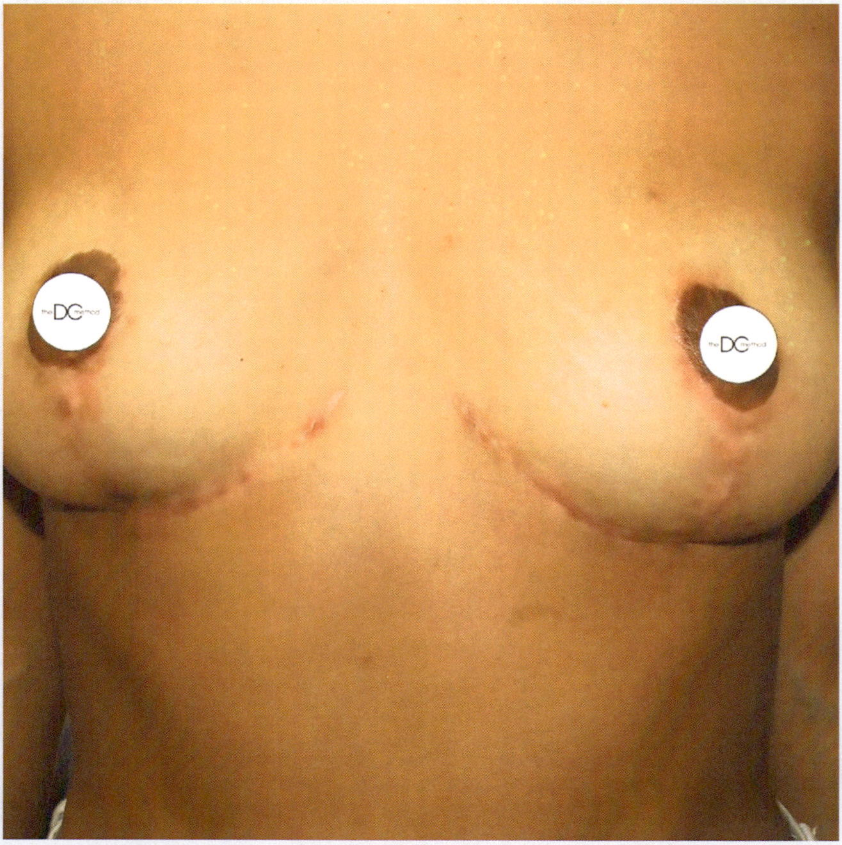

Cesia, 16 Months Post Revision and Keloid Free

Cesia continued, "I'm also buying her products, Scar Food. I restock every time and apply them in the morning and at night."

Scar creams, serums, and specialized soaps are essential in scar treatment. There is a wide range of products available, and I believe this is one of the crucial factors contributing to her success. Honestly, those products are truly remarkable. They nourish the scars, expediting the healing process significantly.

That's my opinion.

I think Linda thought that in a year we were going to be done with it. You know, it's been a year and four months. Literally two days ago, I was talking to her and I sent her a photo so that she can see how they're looking, and I'm going to read the message: she says, "Looks like things are breaking up from the last visit. Honestly, it looks amazing, sweetheart." And I said, "I'm very happy with how the results are showing; I'm finally seeing the light." And she says, "It's been a struggle for sure."

"But I see a light too... Please send me a picture on Monday."

This is what I love about her: she's always on top of everything with her patients.

It's shocking when you see the before and after. Of course, you know, I don't want any scars at all. But if we compare what it was to what it is now, my gosh, I just thought I had to live with the scars for my whole life, you know? I call Linda my angel.

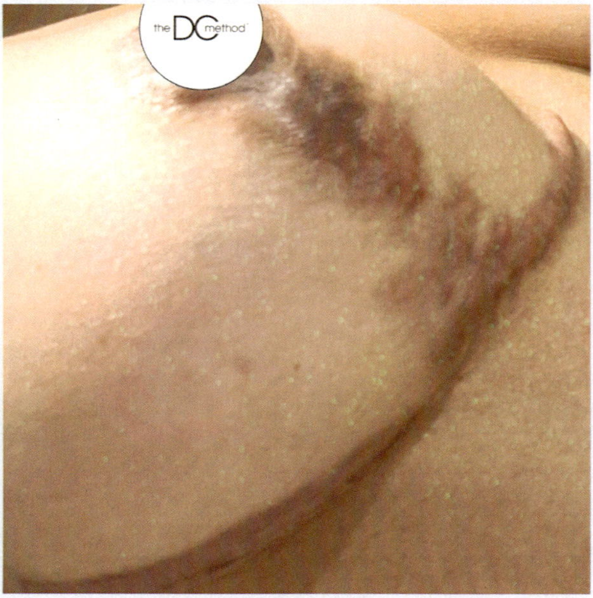

Cesia, Before Keloid Revision

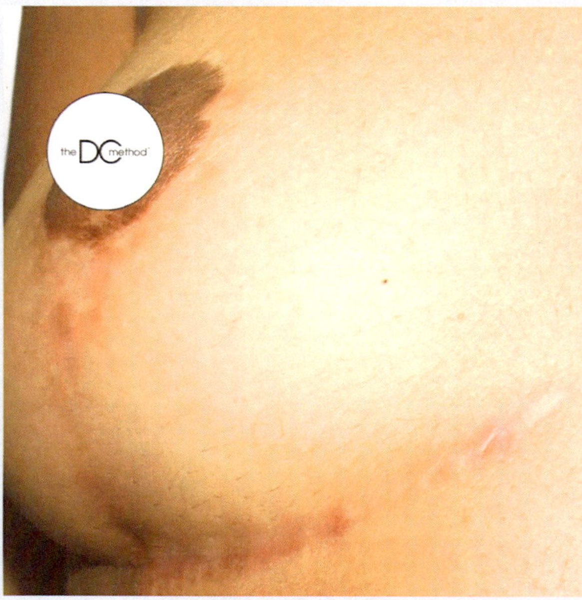

Cesia, 16 Months After Revision: Keloid-Free

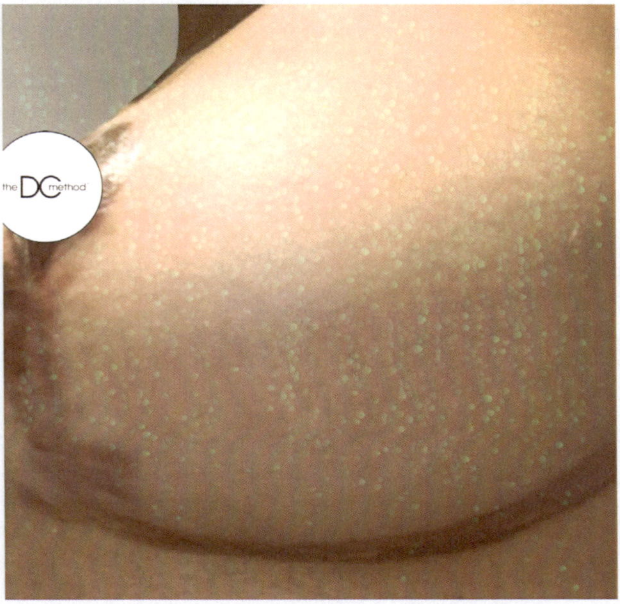

Cesia, Before Keloid Revision

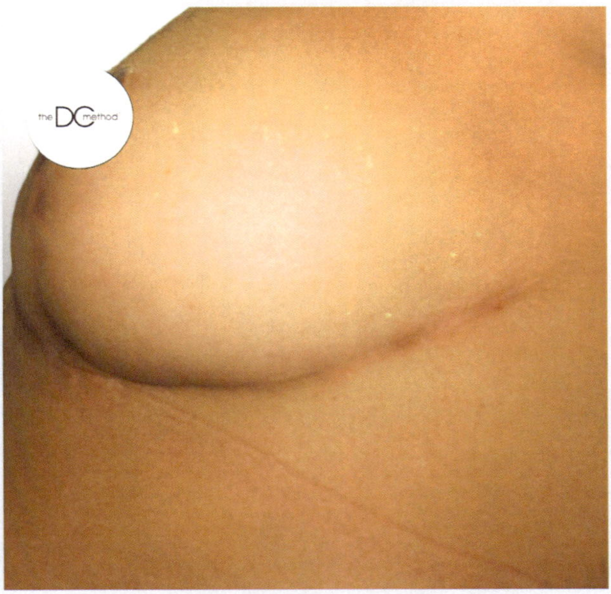

Cesia, 16 Months After Revision. Keloid-Free

SCAR STORY #2 - LIZETTE'S INTERVIEW

My incident actually happened when I was getting ready to graduate from college. I was out at night with a couple of my friends. I didn't know exactly what had happened to me, maybe also due to the shock from it, but I just knew that someone shorter than me had hit me with a bottle across my face. I immediately felt blood dripping. It was a really serious situation.

Something inside me just said, "Walk outside so that I could call 9-1-1." By the time I got to the door, I realized that my face was kind of split open. I could not only put my finger through, but I could also feel the air and my tongue. I could feel everything, and it was bad. When I walked outside, the first thing someone said was, "Don't let her look at herself." It was like a bar brawl, so it wasn't personal. However, there were a lot of people injured.

I probably still cry when I mention the story. Even now, I'm going to have to go back into my memory bank because somehow, I've started kind of forgetting, trying to block the memories. It all happened in April, and it was so bad that I didn't even get to go to my own graduation.

Yeah, it's been a while, but I'm still like a little messed up. I want to cry right now. You know, I really haven't had this conversation. Like, I haven't even discussed it with my psychiatrist. We've talked about everything else, like me as a parent and me dealing with other people. He's even mentioned that one day we'll have to deal with this too because it'll be part of the whole healing journey. But it's really something I don't talk about.

So, I'm in the ambulance. The guy happened to be Hispanic, a Hispanic driver, and he hears me calling my mom. I'm telling her in Spanish, "Hey, something bad happened, but I'm alive..." It's one of the things that I'm still very thankful for. (Lizette is crying now as she recounts the call to her mother.) I was alive! The ambulance guy was like, 'Hey, I'm gonna take you to this place (hospital) because they're known to have the top surgeons, and it looks like you're gonna need it.'

I was truly grateful to be alive, but I felt really messed up; as if my outfit was drenched in blood. It just looked terrible. And I had a feeling that things were going to be tough. Especially because I still consider myself a pretty girl…but back then, I was like really fooling myself and kind of like stuck up. So, the scars really affected me.

Yeah, so we get to the hospital. And I remember having to call my boyfriend and then, like the doctors saying like, 'Oh shit, the boyfriend looks in worse shape than the girlfriend?' I just waited for my mom and family to arrive because my mom had to catch a flight from Miami. This incident happened in Houston. My face had to be stitched up right away. Also, they did an MRI to make sure that none of my bones were broken. And my eye was slid out, like a little bit out of place too.

I was just in total shock, and (after the weekend), I ended up going home. My whole family's with me, and no one's leaving me alone. So the first week, immediately, I'm like trying to figure out what I can do. And most of the doctors are like, "You have to let this heal; we have to see what's going to happen." So they're like, lots of massaging, and you know, minimum talking, minimum smiling.

Just, "let's see how it heals and take it from there." But you know, they were also like, "Just kind of be aware that you're always going to have a scar." So I started kind of learning that: "You're gonna have to deal with this." And that was probably the worst part because I became very reclusive. I didn't want to leave my home. I gained a lot of weight. I came back home and kind of just hid in my old bedroom in my mom's house.

That was April of 2008. And I didn't move back to Miami until the summer. So the good thing about Miami was when I actually started looking for help everybody in Miami is like, of course we can do something about it, we're in like the plastic surgery capital. If there's something we can do, we'll figure it out.' So that was really refreshing because I ended up going to the Miami Institute. It was in the Four Seasons, and I liked the doctor, and he was like, 'What I would do right now is just revise the bottom and, you know, start doing a lot of peels and see where we can go from there?

So my Doctor Gallo did my revision surgery and then It ended up being like a thin line on my face so, you know, I would do hairstyles to hide it and wear makeup. In some lighting, you can barely see it and then in some lighting you can, but when something's directly in your face... (you see it no matter what). I promise you most people are like, 'Liz you know like it's not there…? But that's not how I felt. So I had to keep looking. (Lizette is crying badly and talking with difficulty.) I had to keep looking. It was like there's just no way like this is gonna be like the end, like this. This can't be...

I'm 20-something-years-old, like this just isn't it!

I just kept looking at that's how I found Linda, she's like maybe this method will minimize the way that it looks and we'll try it, you know.

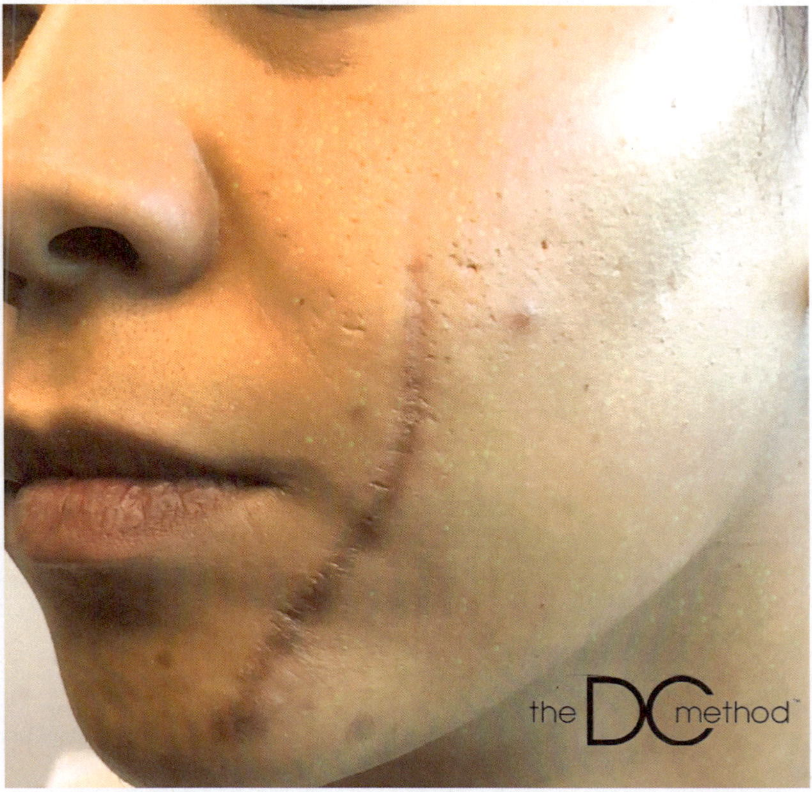

Lizette, Before the DC Method

Lizette continued, "It looks really freakin' good now, but I'm still very hard on myself. It's as good as it's going to get with manmade help. Maybe one day there will be new technology."

You see the outside improvement and you start becoming more comfortable with it because you know how it used to be.

And when something's worse and it's improving, you start accepting it. It feels better. But there's not a point where you're just like, okay, this is normal, or like, I'm back to me.

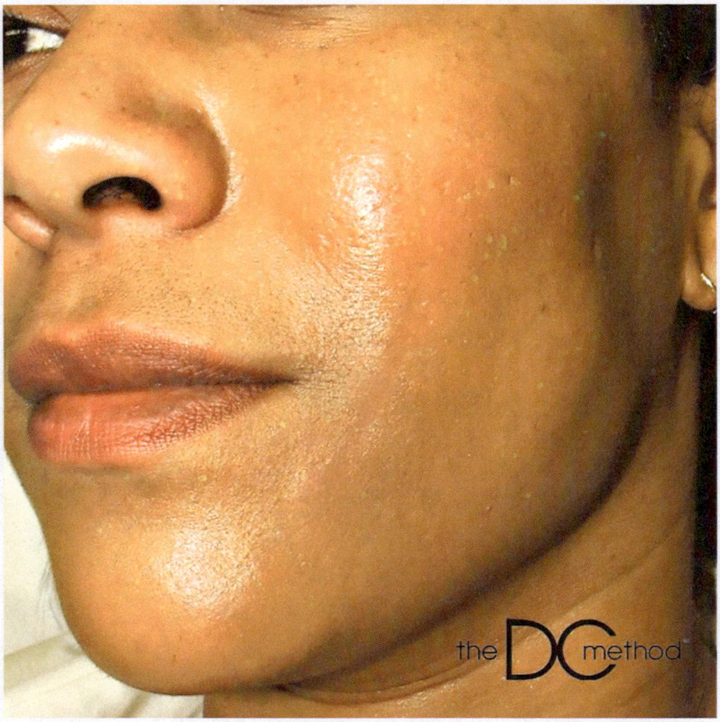

Lizette: 12 Months After We Started Series

Linda: Eight years after her tragic incident, Lizette had endured many surgeries and a daily dose of insecurities and pain. It's not easy to hide facial scars, but also the trauma and PTSD that come along for the ride can be lifelong. I created a 12-month series to revise deep scarring and discoloration.

We made significant aesthetic progress throughout, and in the end, Lizette couldn't believe our results, which far exceeded her expectations. Ironically, the scar has become part of her smile line, which goes unnoticed 90% of the time - well, because she does smile a lot! Seeing a confident Lizette, who now embraces her skin, was an emotional experience, and one I'll always cherish.

PATIENT TIP: "I would say, never stop on your journey. There's definitely going to be some type of help. We can have unrealistic expectations, and at that point, that's when you have to come to terms. But you don't stop looking and you take your time. You know that it's a journey, but there is hope and a chance for improvement... " -

LIZETTE

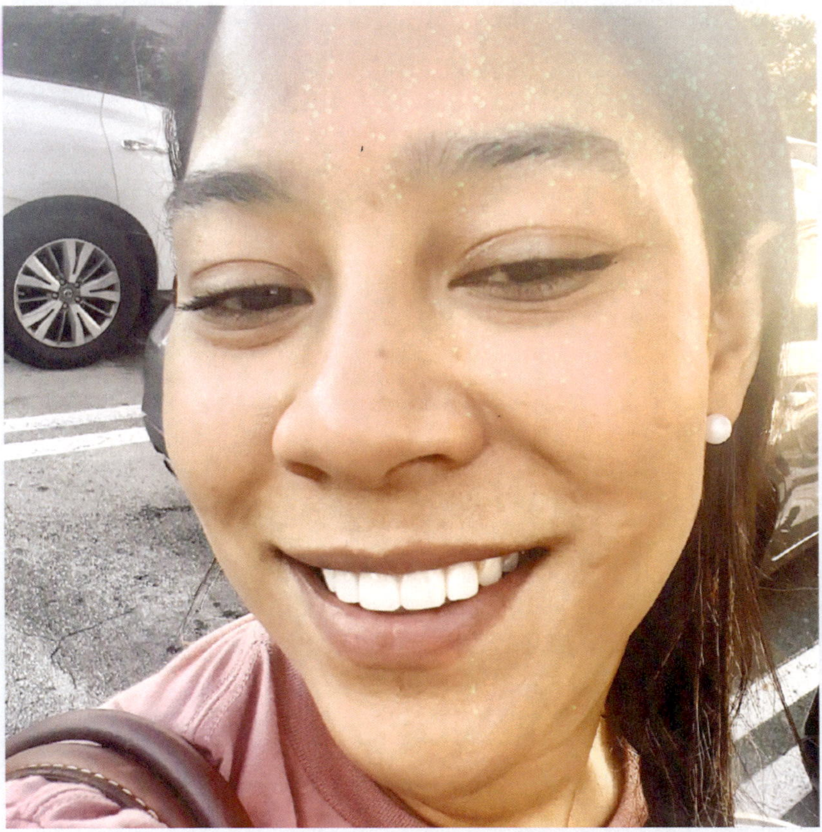

It didn't hinder me professionally, and it didn't hinder my love life. What it did was hinder my personality, my security, and my confidence. It also made me a nicer person; I will say that. I was really full of myself, and I used to do music videos and modeling here and there. So, I was a little arrogant, and this gave me time to kind of humble myself.

One thing I'm definitely thankful for is that I stayed busy, because otherwise I probably would have been super suicidal.

Linda makes you feel comfortable. We ended up bonding, and she genuinely does care about each person as an individual, you know, and that every scar is important to her.

So, not many doctors could say that. She's very special.

Linda: There are many instances throughout the series when I witness my patients transitioning back into real life. They're dating again, wearing open-toe shoes, bathing suits, or more revealing attire, and choosing not to wear makeup to conceal their scars. In those moments, I can't help but think, WOW! Observing my patients with this newfound confidence and seeing them look at themselves in the mirror once more, I know I have fulfilled my duty!

PRO TIP: The DC Method team is always available to answer questions and provide expert advice. Don't hesitate to call 866-SCARTLK if you need information or just someone to listen.

CHAPTER 3

DUNN WITH SCARS: THE DC METHOD IS BORN

WHAT IS THE DC METHOD?

My name is Linda Dunn-Carter, and my trademark brand, **The DC Method**, began in 2006. Since then, **The DC Method**™ has empowered me to perform more than 65,000 scar and corrective skin care procedures, gaining global recognition in the field of scar revision. You may be wondering, what exactly is **The DC Method**™? The "DC" stands for me, Dunn-Carter, and "The Method" represents a series of time-specific protocols that transform old scars into new skin and guide scars towards complete healing. I refer to this approach as the "less-traveled road."

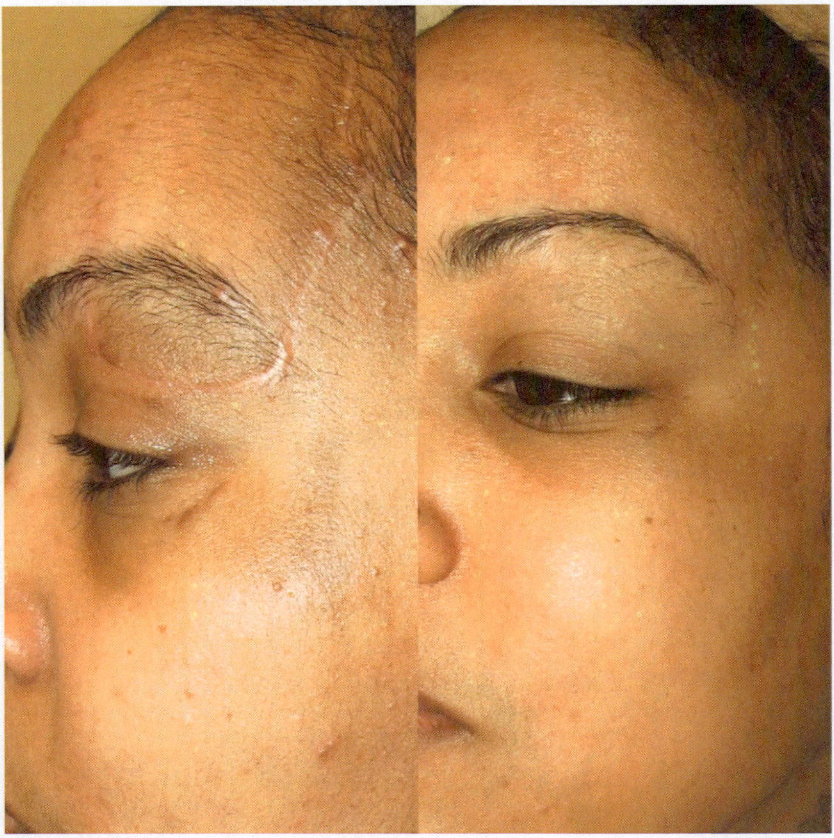

Knife Wounds: Before and After the DC Method

It felt like destiny was calling when I took a class called "Scar Relaxation" back in 2006. Immediately, I thought, "Why only relax the scar? Why not fix it? Why not repair the scar so it becomes invisible?" It was like a light bulb went off in my head - my "ah-hah" moment! I had just received my Aesthetician License to work in skincare, and a few months later, I enrolled in a PMU (Permanent Makeup) Institute, where I obtained multiple Certifications, including Areola Tattooing and Scar Relaxation. I was immediately intrigued by scars, and I knew right then that's what I wanted to do - fix scars! However,

I didn't know how that would play out since there were no schools to teach me scar revision. So, I set out to teach myself. I basically needed the answer to one question: "If I were a scar, what would it take to fix me, inside and out?" I spent hundreds of hours researching medical journals and attending medical webinars - anything I could get my hands on. I compiled all the data I could find relating to scars, the healing process, and different skin and scar types.

Ultimately, this would result in many different protocols, where each would hand off to the other in order to reprogram scars, create new skin, and achieve the most natural results possible.

My theory: In order to make new skin, I must first injure the skin or scar by abrading the superficial layer and breaking bands of tethered scar tissue underneath. This provides the necessary information for the skin to transform into new tissue. The steps to follow are equally important, where key nutrients such as stem cells, peels, and peptides are infused into the abraded tissue. This promotes rapid cell turnover and encourages new tissue growth. As the skin heals over the next 30 days it creates a layer of dead skin that is removed making way for the new tissue that ultimately creates the change in the way the appearance of the scars look over time. These steps are time-sensitive and repetitive, and achieving the best possible results would require several months. The protocols would need to be modified during each visit based on the patient's healing progress. Knowledgeable skin assessments are crucial for moving forward.

I was eager to put my newfound knowledge into play and started my journey of case studies one after another. It was incredible to see so many people volunteer to be case studies and even more incredible to see major changes in as little as one month when they returned for their next visit. I knew I was onto something great.

With the mounting positive evidence, The DC Method™ was born. Since then, I have documented all my cases to track the power of The DC Method™ techniques.

Although it's a proven method, rebirthing skin is not instant gratification. The patient's commitment to the process is paramount and can take 6-18 months, depending on the severity of their scars, to make them less visible to the eye.

SPREADING THE WORD

I opened my first office in Sedona, AZ, in 2006 and quickly moved to a larger market in Scottsdale, AZ. It wasn't easy launching a brand-new idea in a market that wasn't established or in demand like it is today. Still, I believed my method would change lives and industry standards and aggressively forged forward. Those beliefs have since come to fruition.

Demand for The DC Method™ continued to grow, and I expanded into larger demographics, including Miami, FL, in 2014. The road in Miami was briefly bumpy as chaos in my personal life (and even brief homelessness) challenged my will to persevere, but with God's good graces, I overcame the setbacks. Today, my credentials speak loudly and proudly. Currently, I'm a licensed aesthetician in six states.

Since my move to Miami in 2014, I've expanded my clinics to four major cities: Houston, TX; Miami Beach, FL; NYC; and Atlanta, GA.

Patients are seen on a rotating basis, and nothing could be more rewarding.

Another passion of mine is teaching The **DC Method**™. This passion has led me to open my training center in Miami Beach, FL, called "Scar School by The **DC Method**." At this school, we provide scar revision education, scar plan protocols, theory, and practical hands-on skills to industry professionals who share our passion for fixing scars and changing lives. But I haven't stopped there.

My latest endeavors include a full line of scar care products called "Scar Food by The DC Method™" and my newest completed goal, a franchise namely **ScarFixClinic**™. My franchise business offers a complete turnkey clinic to qualified franchisees in all 50 US states and US territories. These additional clinics should allow even more patients to find the urgent scar care they need. When I'm not busy caring for scar patients, it's my passion to lobby for legislation that will set more specific regulatory standards within the Body Art Industry. From what I've personally seen and treated, there's an urgent need to inform consumers in order to prevent unnecessary injuries and scarring that are taking place every day within the industry.

The first step in each and every scar journey is offering reliable information and giving patients hope. This information can be found on multiple social media platforms, blogs, websites, news media, as well as my podcast

"Dunn With The Scar." It's one more layer of education where consumers can learn tips about the dos and don'ts of scar care.

RESULTS THAT SPEAK VOLUMES

Patients tend to be visual; you can talk all day about what you do, but *photos are what they want to see*. They want to see realistic results, and I'm very honest and transparent about the expectations I can fulfill. Patients deserve to be walked through the process of the series on every level - the what, when, why, where, and how of the series. I preach total dedication and follow-through to The DC Method™ team. We constantly strive to build trust with our patients and rapport with our industry peers.

For me, growth means continuously developing expertise and advanced skills in scar repair, which result in consistently high levels of success, even in the most complex cases. We have reached a stage where there is no longer a need to reject anyone. The DC Method can effectively address any type of scar or skin issue to a greater extent than what was achievable in the early years of my career.

ONE-STOP SHOPPING FOR SCAR CARE

It was important to grow to a level of becoming a one-stop shop for our patients. This involved creating my scar repair product line, **Scar Food**. Combined with physical treatments, these **Scar Food** products have a synergistic effect: They help to soothe scars while also speeding up the growth of new tissue and the healing of both old and new scars. My **Scar Food** line of products also brought more attention to wound care. **Scar Food** customers often sought advice or referrals for scar treatment through **The DC Method**™. So, adding the availability of a scar product line was a win-win combination for the patients. Having a product that you use on your own patients to get top-notch results gives the patients even more trust.

They are confident that these products truly target their scars.

They know not only that we endorse the products, but that we actually created them!

RATING PATIENT SATISFACTION

Even as The DC Method™ and the Scar Food line have grown, patient satisfaction has remained a preeminent focus. Our patients show an extremely high level of satisfaction and success in using Scar Food Products in between their in-office visits.

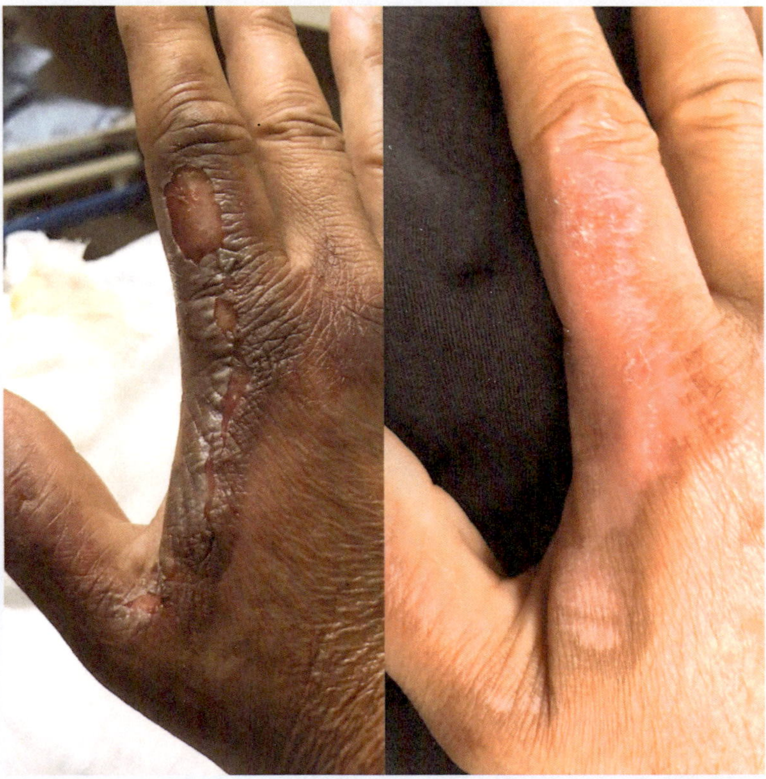

Grease Burn: 2.5 Weeks on Scar Food

SCAR STORY #3 - MIRI'S INTERVIEW

Miri: "So, I had a breast lift in Miami, Florida, with a well-known and highly regarded surgeon. He had like a lot of followers on Instagram. And he also posted a lot of pictures. And it looked like his technique was nice. There was like minimal scarring on every picture that he showed, and that's why I decided to go with him. The first time I ever met up with him was like the day before surgery. I told him like the size breast that I wanted, you know, like a full C. He said,
"Okay, that's fine."

WHAT MY DOCTOR DIDN'T TELL ME: "The doctor didn't mention any risks or anything; he just came on the day of the surgery and drew on me. He did his markings and then we went back to the operating room. He didn't even tell me how long the surgery would take.

"So they had me go back the next day and he was not available to see me. I think I saw his nurse and she said:

"Everything looks good." When I came back the next day (day 3) he took off the tapes from over my incisions. There were like blisters. And to me because, you know, I'm a Surgical Tech, to me it looked like necrosis.

At that point, he [the Doctor] was talking to his nurses, and he was saying: "Well, how did this happen?" He's like: "Did you guys put the tape on too tight?" That's what he said. He kind of went to grab a pair of pickups (surgical tool) and just kind of took off the blisters.

"And then he's like, 'Was I a smoker?' And I said, "No," and I said, "I mean, I smoke like hookah and I vape from time to time but like, I don't smoke cigarettes, anything like that." And then he sent me to get hyperbaric treatments (treatment in an oxygen chamber to help the skin heal.) It was like five days with the extra oxygen care on the wound and then I came back to see him. And he's like: 'Okay, you should be good. You're not gonna lose your breast. You're not gonna lose your nipple. You're gonna be good?

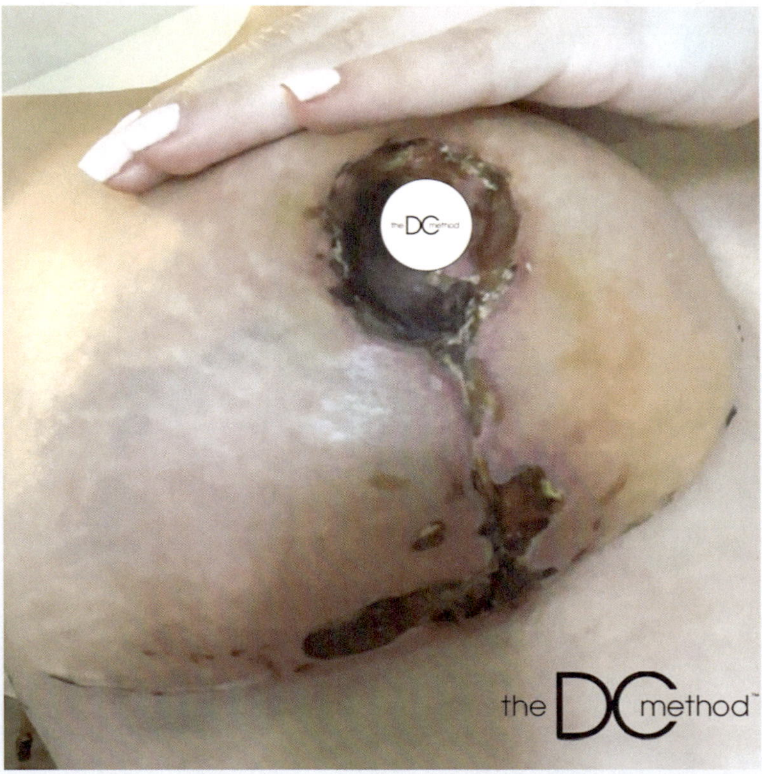

Miri, After Hyperbaric Treatment

After that, I came back home [to Louisiana], and from there, I was pretty much on my own.

I wasn't able to talk to my surgeon anymore. I was just following up with his nurses. I called them and said, "I need help; you need to help me with these treatments!" And they said:

"No! What really upset me was that she (the nurse) told me that this was my fault because I was a smoker...and that was why I got the necrosis. So, I said, "Well, I'm going to find a lawyer..." After that, they transferred me to his PA, his Physician's Assistant, on their app. What made me more upset was how they handled it after what happened."

Maybe they could have been more helpful, you know? They just don't care. Like, they really don't care.

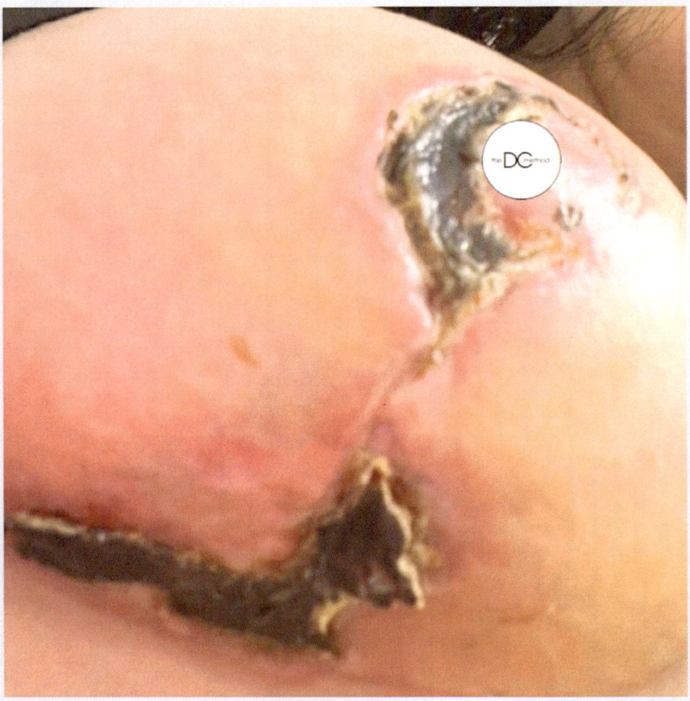

Miri, Healing Slowly....

WHAT MY DOCTOR DIDN'T TELL ME.

"There's a lot the doctors don't say. Like, for example, how they don't close the incisions themselves after surgery. I knew there were risks but with what I was paying I expected he would close the incision and he didn't. They used heat to close my incision; they used a tool called a Bovie. I know about the tool because I work in surgery as an Operation Technician. But also, the Dr. at the Hyperbaric Center confirmed it: he actually told me the damage was caused by too much heat...**Miri.**"

PATIENT TIP: "Just because something seems good on the internet doesn't mean that it is. Make sure that they're going to have good patient care after the surgery and that they are not just after your money. – *Miri.*"

Miri: I was able to find a doctor back in New Orleans, where I live, who specializes in wound care - Dr. Paul Harch, MD. He administered more hyperbaric treatments, which proved to be really helpful. Although I was relieved that I was ok, but the scars were terrible. I was so depressed. I cried every day.

Juan Juan (Mir's husband): We have to pay around $4,000 out of pocket for the additional hyperbaric treatment...every week Miri went. She was so depressed and crying every day. It was like that until we went to see Linda...Linda Dunn-Carter in Houston, Texas

Miri: So, I think I saw her (Linda Dunn-Carter) on Instagram. And, you know, I contacted her. My wound had just recently closed. So, she said to wait a little while longer before coming to her. And I did. And then she made a plan for me.

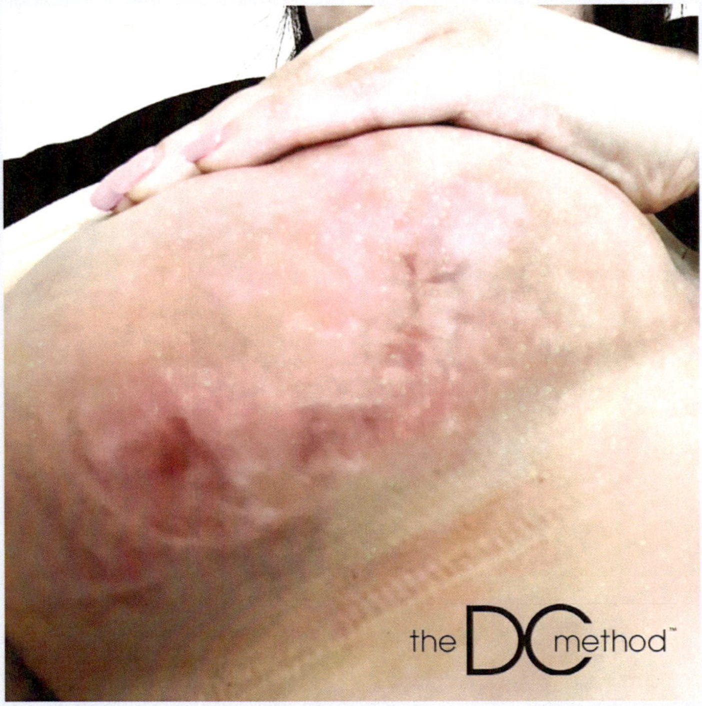

Miri's Scar: When We Started the DC Method

She said she was gonna do the best she could; and she said that maybe it would be a 90% (improvement). And she did it.

I mean, the size of this gapping scar that I had, compared to like, what I have left is like, barely noticeable.

The treatment was about ten months. I finished around March of 2023.

Juan Juan- (**Miri's** husband) We had to drive to Houston — six and a half hours each way, once a month. But after the first couple of visits Miri was coming back. You could tell; Linda was showing her she was going to be ok.

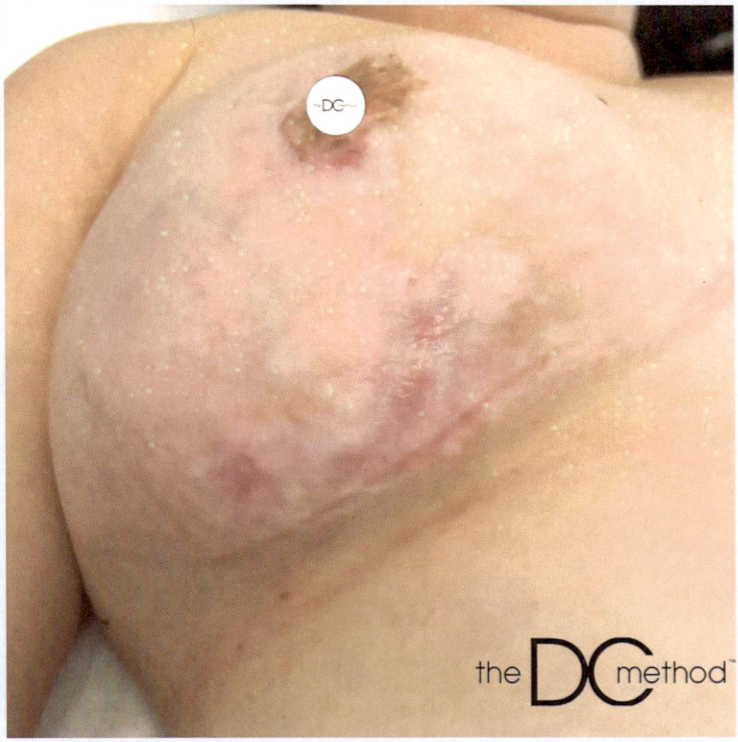

Miri, After a Few Visits

Linda: A straightforward breast lift procedure ended in disaster for Miri. She had suffered months of post-op complications to her right breast. Hyperbaric treatments helped to heal her gaping wounds, which ultimately left terrible scars behind. Unfortunately, contrary to her surgeon's statement, she did end up losing more than half of her areola and nipple, which I transformed to near perfection.

I recommended a ten-month plan, and her mood began to improve almost immediately. Miri had hope and was finally on the path to healing, inside and out. Her results after ten months were nearly perfect, and her self-esteem is back for good. I couldn't be prouder of her and her husband's commitment to the process and the results it brought her!

Miri: You know, once I got to her, Linda helped me, not only on the outside, but she helped me bring my self-esteem back up. I felt much better. You know, just having someone who actually cares about what she does. Yeah, I'm very grateful for Linda. She changed my life!

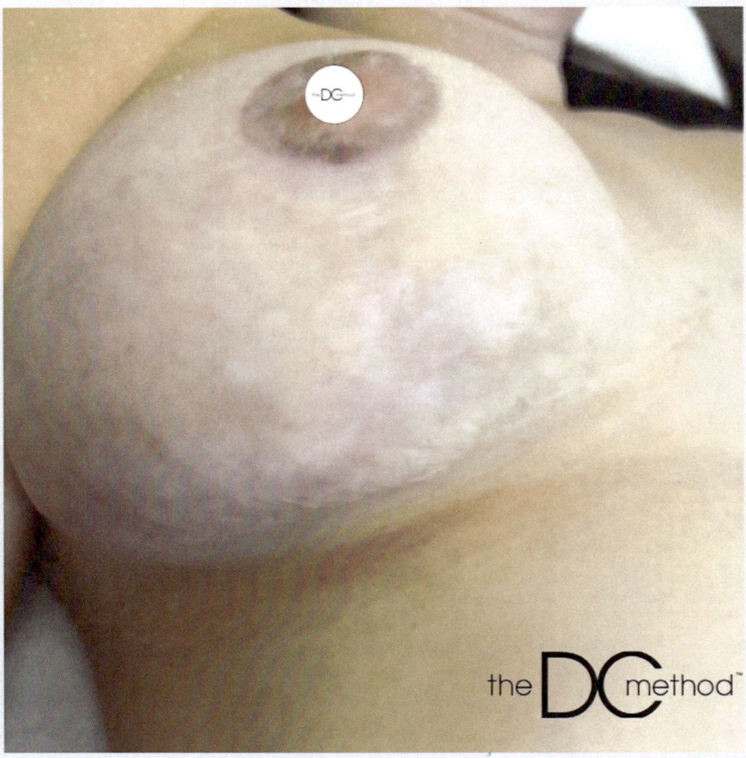

Miri's Final Results!

SCAR STORY #4 - J'ADORE'S INTERVIEW

I've had a scar all my life: I was burned as a child. I tried several different methods, I even had a tattoo to try and conceal the burns on my hand, but that did not work out well.

So then, I had a few laser sessions to attempt removal. During that process, they actually burned my pigment worse, causing it to turn white, plus leaving behind a lot more scarring. It was so ugly and noticeable that I was definitely self-conscious about its appearance.

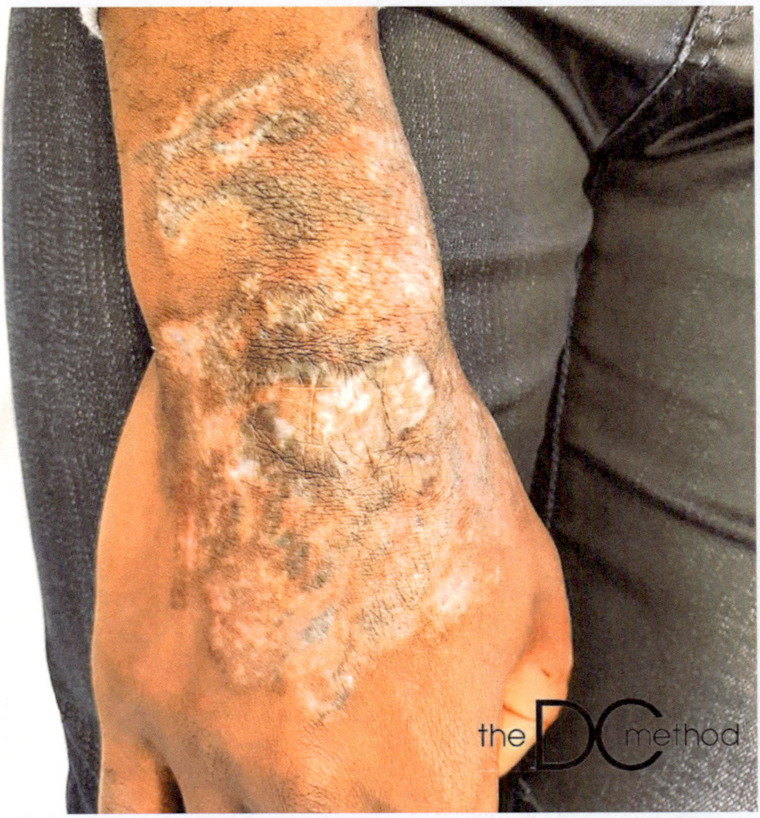

J'Adore Before the DC Method

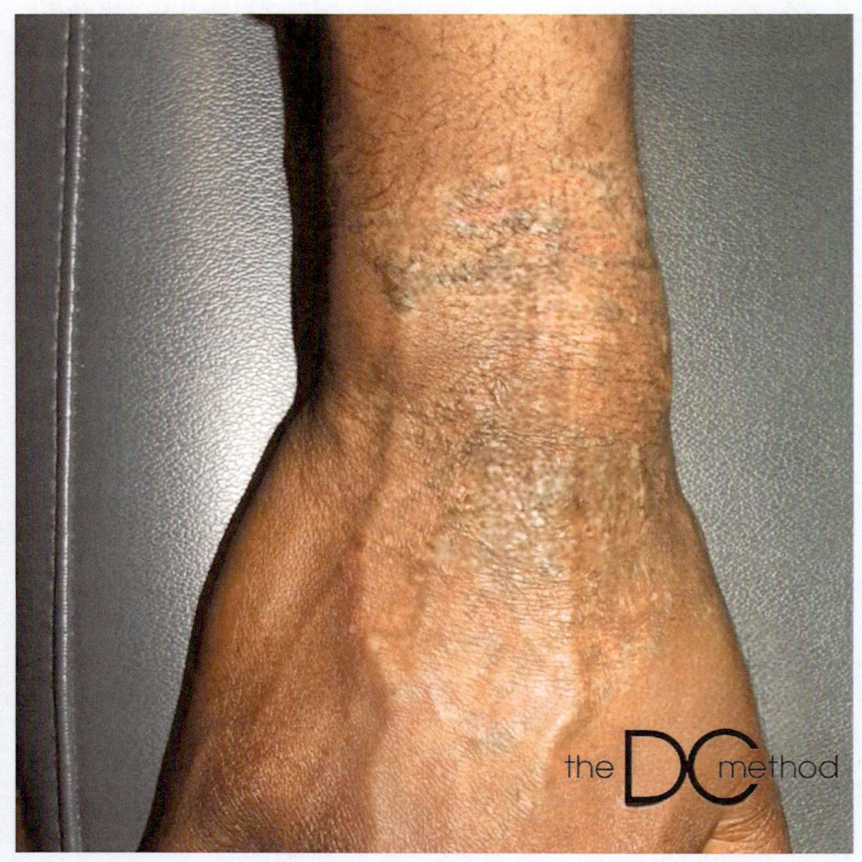

J'Adore After 6 Months: The DC Method.

Later, as an adult, I also had a rhinoplasty that left me with a scar along my nostrils. I didn't even want to look in the mirror. It really destroyed my confidence - especially in my work as a nurse practitioner when I was up close with my patients.

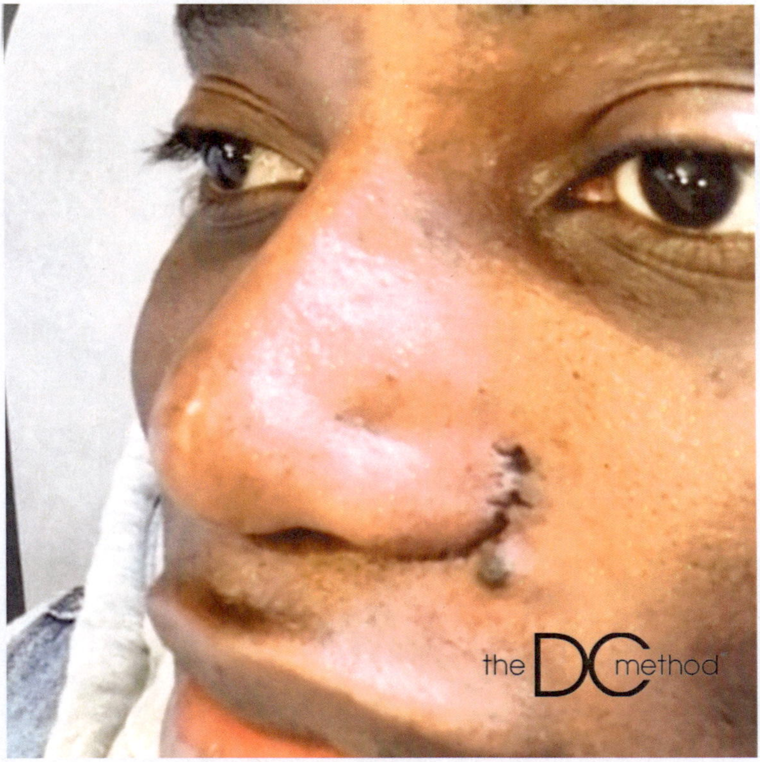

J'Adore Before the DC Method

I went on the internet and started doing some research on different ways to manage this surgical scar because I just didn't want to go through another procedure to revise it.

During my search, I came across The DC Method and Linda Dunn-Carter. When we first met, we connected instantly. Ever since then, I have had nothing but good things to say about my experience. My scars are behind me. I no longer look in the mirror at my burns or my nostrils and feel self-conscious about how I look. My self-esteem is back, and I know the inside and outside scars are all behind me. That's all thanks to Linda.

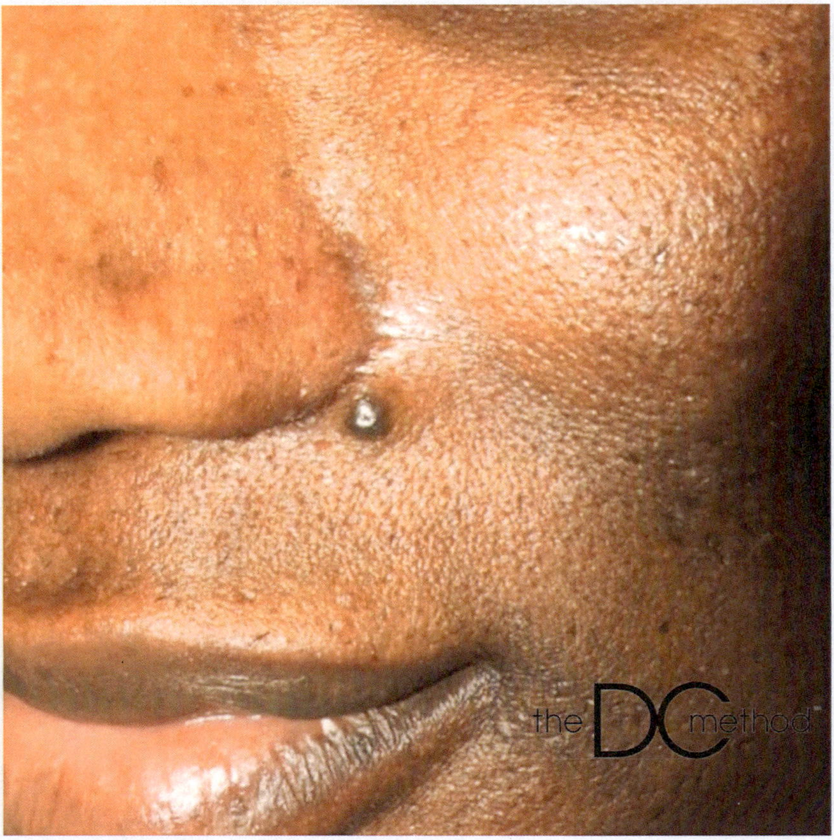

J'Adore After the DC Method

WHAT MY DOCTOR DIDN'T TELL ME. "You know, I always tell my patients, and this is something I learned: you have to interview your surgeon the same way you go and someone interviews you for a job. You have to interview your surgeon and make sure that they're prudent, make sure the surgery is something they specialize in, because anyone can put out ads and say, oh tummy tuck, or liposuction ... here this is what it costs. But how many of those cases have those doctors actually done? How long have they actually been doing it for? It's all about honesty and openness." J'Adore Mattis

Linda: J'Adore came to me after undergoing a rhinoplasty revision, which was basically a botched attempt to correct his scar issues. Unfortunately, it only made them worse, resulting in deep holes on both sides of his nostrils. Additionally, he had a bad burn on his hand from laser tattoo removal, which I also addressed. My ten-month treatment plan to repair his scars has completely raised his self-esteem and restored his confidence. Now, he has no problem being close up when talking to people, without the fear that they are staring at his nose or hand. It was truly a blessing to be able to restore his beautiful aesthetic appearance. J'Adore genuinely cares for his patients, so it was especially rewarding to be there for him.

PATIENT TIP: "I work as a Nurse Practitioner, and I can enthusiastically refer my patients who have scars - from the tiniest to the most humongous. I don't think that there's any scar that Linda cannot tackle." *– J'Adore Mattis.*

Linda: My biggest takeaway is how rewarding it is to change lives by significantly repairing scars that are debilitating and cause self-esteem issues. My ultimate mission is to give my patients back their self-esteem and allow them to live their best lives. I believe this is my true God-given purpose: to fulfill this mission and heal my patients one scar at a time.

The DC Method™ team is always available to answer questions and provide referrals. Don't hesitate to call our hotline 866-SCARTLJ if you need advice, information, or just someone to listen.

CHAPTER 4
RESEARCH AND THE ALL-IMPORTANT CONSULTATION

PART 1: DON'T FORGET THE RESEARCH!

WHERE DO I EVEN START?

There are many different ways to research a surgeon. I'm going to guide you through some of the best resources and some of my favorite go-to platforms The Internet and social media. First of all, you'll want to target surgeons who specialize in the specific surgical procedure you are considering. Looking for a specific procedure will narrow your research considerably.

For cosmetic surgeries that are not covered by insurance, you will have a wide variety of surgeons. If your insurance company requires a referral for Other kinds of surgery - heart procedures or orthopedic procedures, for example - may limit your choices. Regardless, it is crucial to conduct thorough research. The location and credentials of your surgeon are important, as well as the number of procedures they have performed and their success rate. Additionally, the quality and availability of post-operative care are critical in minimizing scar complications. If you prioritize finding the best cost-cutting deal over these essential factors, you may be making a risky and unwise decision.

> **PRO TIP**: "It is highly recommended to choose a local surgeon in case there are post-surgical complications. Many surgeons are hesitant to fix problems from a previous surgeon's work. Scouting for a surgeon at a moment's notice when things go wrong is very stressful and costly." – *Linda Dunn-Carter*

If you have surgery in another state or abroad and suffer post-surgical complications, most surgeons in your area will turn you away simply because it's not their work. At that point, your only recourse might be the local hospital to treat your immediate condition and not anything else. You'll recover, but you'll lose the option for more meticulous treatment that perhaps the original surgeon could have provided.

My bestie said the surgeon was great.

You might know someone who raves about a successful surgery from a particular surgeon, but there are important questions you should ask yourself when considering a referral like this - or any surgeon for that matter. Remember, no two people heal the same, nor have the same skin type or color. So what a friend or relative might have experienced is not necessarily what you will experience. Even though a referral from a trusted friend can be reassuring, we all need to do our homework!

If you are tempted to go with a referral, ask yourself, "What are my risks?"

Are you having the same type of surgery?

Are your circumstances the same, such as body type, skin type, and inherited traits?

What is this surgeon's overall success rate with this specific procedure?

Do they receive high praise from former patients?

PRO TIP: "Just because a surgeon was successful with one patient doesn't make them the right surgeon for you. Your risk profile might be totally different."
– Linda Dunn-Carter

WHAT TO LOOK FOR

It's only natural for surgeons to put their best foot forward.

They want your business. You can assume that the photos you see of their procedures are likely to show their best outcomes and not the complications. So, here are some key questions that will help you examine credentials and what a surgeon can actually do for you:

Is your prospective surgeon board-certified? It's critical to have a board-certified surgeon perform your surgery. To check your surgeon's credentials, you can visit the American Board of Medical Specialties website, abms.org, and search for your surgeon online.

Have any malpractice claims been filed by your surgeon's state medical board?

What do former patients say? For example, do the patients mention scars? Do they mention complications? Do they talk about the quality and availability of aftercare?

If you haven't researched this kind of topic before, you may find an overwhelming amount of information available online. Let's review a convenient list of some of my favorite go-to platforms.

SCARS: WHAT DRS. DIDN'T TELL THEM. Would you believe that 90 percent of my patients confirm being under-informed about critical details of their surgery, such as the quantity and placement of their scars, and the aftercare?

MY SHORTLIST OF THE BEST RESOURCES

Facebook Support Groups:
To find support groups related to specific surgeries, such as "Breast Lift Groups" or "Brachioplasty Groups," simply enter the surgery type in the search bar. This will lead you to numerous groups where people openly discuss their experiences with the surgery and the surgeons involved. Personally, I find this platform to be one of my favorites. However, in order to access the valuable information shared within these groups, you will need to request to join and be approved.

Within these groups, you will find open discussions that cover both the positive and negative aspects of the surgeries. Members who have already undergone the surgery or are considering it share real-time photos, details about their recovery process, and the names of the surgeons they used. Most importantly, they also discuss the physical and emotional scars left behind and the different stages of healing. It is worth noting that some of the information shared may be encouraging, while other details may discourage you from pursuing the surgery. Nevertheless, it is important to hear the honest opinions and experiences of real people, both the good and the bad.

It is rare to find a practitioner with a 100% positive review, and it is important to remember that some negative reviews may be unwarranted and come from individuals who are simply angry in general. However, with careful consideration and by using your own judgment, along with the compiled information from these groups, you can make an informed decision.

PRO TIP: "It's a process, so be patient and don't give up easily. All of this research and education ultimately impact the results in a positive way."
– Linda Dunn-Carter

INSTAGRAM: Search for the type of surgery or hashtag it.
This will take you to tons of pages displaying different information about your type of surgery. The volume of material can be a bit overwhelming, but don't let it deter you.

You can also search for the surgeon's name. Beware that Instagram or X accounts can present a questionable sense of reality because most pages will show successful surgeries that appear flawless. Consumers shouldn't assume their case will look like the results in these handpicked photos.

> **PRO TIP**: "Nowadays a lot of patients obtain information from the internet and social media. However, despite having access to a wealth of information, they may not fully comprehend what is most suitable for their specific skin types.
>
> Hopefully, by the time they leave their surgeon's office, they're better informed. In plastic surgery, the scars are a large part of the final result, and patient education is important." *– Dr. Pamela Brownlee, Plastic and Reconstructive Surgeon"*

REAL SELF: Use this platform to research surgeons and types of surgery. This site is another personal favorite of mine. You will need to sign up to navigate through the website', but it's totally worth it. This site functions a little differently because it features questions posted by people who have experienced complications from surgery or injury. These questions are then answered by board-certified surgeons who provide recommendations for treatment or guidance on how to proceed in a given situation. Additionally, you will have access to real-time photos showcasing progress

Complications, and success. Typing in a surgeon's name will also lead to reviews and any interaction they may have had on the site.

This platform has everything and is a fabulous source of educational information.

> **PRO TIP**: "Post-care reviews by patients are often the best indicator of how a surgeon cares for you once they have collected your money and performed the surgery." – *Linda Dunn-Carter*

GOOGLE REVIEWS: Type in the name of the surgeon you are considering. This will provide you with additional testimony regarding their expertise, skills, and outcomes from real patients. Post-care reviews can reveal an astonishing lack of aftercare from some surgeons who suddenly have no time for their patients. Again, it's rare to find a 100% review on any practitioner, and sometimes reviews left are unwarranted from angry individuals in general. You can easily identify them. Keep your radar on alert for the beeping red flags to make a full assessment.

Never forget, 'it's a job interview

An all-inclusive experience with your prospective surgeon(s) will include their attention to detail during your upcoming consultation. As the interviewer, you'll have a chance to observe their bedside manners, their commitment to answering questions, their apparent honesty about "what-if" complications, and their availability for critical aftercare.

PART II THE ALL-IMPORTANT CONSULTATION

Congratulations! You have done your research and decided on a specific candidate to perform your surgery. Now it's time for the consultation. This is the final and most important step, and it's where you determine if you will ultimately select this surgeon. So, guess what, most surgeons won't just voluntarily offer up a wealth of information. It will be up to you to ask away. My patients have been a very good source for me to compile an extensive list of questions that will help you prepare better than they had.

Remember, surgery is a big deal, and when investing in surgery or scar revision, it's not uncommon to have multiple consultations before coming to a decision. You'll want a surgeon who has your best interests at heart, so consulting with several surgeons to compare notes can be an extremely wise move.

PRO TIP: "Not only are consultations and surgical plans important, but they are also legally required."
– Linda Dunn-Carter

It is highly rare, but if a surgeon refuses a consultation, he or she should not be considered. Even with a consultation, more than 90% of my patients have verified that they were underinformed during their consultation, especially when it came to aftercare. This is why I have prepared a list of questions that will not only benefit your end results but will also give you peace of mind.

WHAT MY DOCTOR DIDN'T TELL ME.

Post-op Post-operative surgical surprises are simply unacceptable, and the key to avoiding them is to ask a lot of questions. For instance, I had a patient who underwent a skinny Brazilian Butt Lift that required liposuction. To our astonishment, after the surgery, we discovered a total of seventeen entry points on this petite individual. It's worth noting that she wasn't even overweight before the procedure. When I inquired whether she was aware of the number of scars she would have, she replied, "No." The discussion regarding the number and placement of scars on her body had never taken place. Neither the patient thought to inquire nor did the surgeon volunteer the information. Personally, if I had known that I would end up with seventeen small incisions, each leaving a visible scar, I would have emphatically declined. What is most troubling to me is that these kinds of outrageous oversights occur on a regular basis.

THE ELEPHANT IN THE ROOM

Surgeons don't want to scare you by talking about scar risks, but unfortunately, scars are a crucial topic to cover. I mean, you are going to be cut, so there is a 100% chance you will have a scar to live with after the surgery. You are entitled to an answer for every question you ask during your consultation. This applies to questions after the procedure as well. Some people might feel intimidated by doctors and don't want to overstep or insinuate anything by asking certain pointed questions. You must remember that you are basically interviewing your surgeon for a job, and that job requires cutting on you! Prior to surgery, you have 100% control. The more thorough you are in asking questions, the less chance there will be of unpleasant surprises. Also, if you don't understand their answer, ask again.

If you don't get that warm, fuzzy feeling during the consultation, or don't like how the questions were answered - maybe you felt rushed or they skirted around the questions - then believe the red flags and consider another provider. You should feel completely comfortable with your provider during the entire consultation! Period.

PAYING FOR YOUR CONSULT

The cost of a consultation varies or can even be free. If there is a fee involved, ask if that fee is credited towards the service. The important thing is to be prepared with all your questions before your consultation and ask the surgeon or staff if there is anything you will need to bring with you to your appointment. You will definitely want to bring a notepad or smartphone to take notes in person while your memory is fresh.

PRO TIP: "Take your own before photos from the front and both sides of the area that will be cut, or the existing scar, to keep for your personal records."
– Linda Dunn-Carter

QUESTIONS FOR YOUR SURGEON

I have included a comprehensive list of questions as a reference. You can choose from those that appear most relevant to your situation, your surgery, and your follow-up care or scar revision.

- How many procedures or surgeries have they performed like yours and on the same type of skin?
- Are there before and after photos of the same surgery on my skin type? If there are only a few or none at all, should I reconsider?
- What is required pre-op or procedure? Are there any dietary guidelines to gain or lose weight? Is blood work necessary? Is there a specific home care routine that needs to be followed?
- Where will the surgery be performed?
- Who will be performing the surgery? This might sound obvious, but you will not know if an intern or resident will perform the actual procedure, so it's actually an extremely valid question.
- Who will be in the room during my surgery?
- Who will be doing the suturing? This is a very important step since the quality of your sutures will have a dramatic impact on how you will heal and the outcome of your scars. Experience is key when it comes to suturing. Many times, this critical role is handed off to another person.
- What kind of sutures will be used? If you have issues with spitting sutures that your body rejects, then what's the alternative? Nylon sutures, liquid sutures, or?
- What if your body rejects the dissolvable sutures?
- Will the aftercare cover that, or will the surgeon be available for assistance?
- Will there be drains? How many? How long? Where will they be placed?
- How many surgeries will be performed on the day of your surgery?
- Where will you be in that lineup? If your surgery is complex and you are last, ask to reschedule on a different day.

Remember, surgeons are human and can become fatigued if pushed to the maximum. Some states limit the number of surgeries they can perform in a day.

- Where exactly on my body will the scars be located?
- How long will the scars be?
- Where will the scars be placed on the body? This is important if you're wanting the scars to be discreet and covered by certain clothing or swimsuits.
- What if there are complications like an open incision, infection, or worse? What do you do? Is this information covered in the Aftercare section?
- What if I have a keloid afterwards? Will Kenalog injections be included?
- If not, how much extra are they?
- How often would they be needed?
- What is the revision policy if something isn't right the first time? Is it free or not?
- What is the best and worst-case scenario regarding any healing or surgical complications, in their opinion? This could be a question based on your skin type, if you heal poorly with keloids or are prone to hypertrophic scarring. Surgeons should be able to give you these scenarios.
- What are the risks during and after the kind of surgery or procedure you are receiving?
- Are photos or videos taken in the surgical room or at any time during the procedures? If so, you will need to sign a form giving consent.
- Request that photos be taken immediately after surgery, before you are taped up. These photos are especially important for validating the work. Incisions can become compromised during

tape removal, so seeing them beforehand provides peace of mind.

- How do you obtain your before, during, and after photos? They serve as a record and will be useful in case anything goes awry.
- If applicable, what will you be wearing or not wearing during surgery? For instance, if you are undergoing facial surgery, will you be wearing a gown or will you be draped? This has been a recurring concern based on the experiences of several of my patients.
- What can be expected in the first month after surgery in terms of healing? It's important for you to understand the phases that your incision will go through after surgery. Will it bleed? Swell?

Bruise? What level of pain should you expect and for how long?

- Would compression garments be advisable, and if so, what type?
- What about lymphatic massages afterward? How many? Cost?
- What would a good scenario look like after a month?
- What would a worst-case scenario look like after a month?
- When can you go back to work? What about exercising and driving?
- What is the cost?
- What is included in the cost? Are post-op appointments included? What is included in those appointments? This is particularly important if you are traveling to see the provider. Is the overnight stay included? Is there a nurse on watch? You get the message.
- Does the provider offer financing?

Just be aware that not all questions will be answered by the surgeon themselves. There could be process or payment questions that the patient coordinator may have knowledge of, so make certain these other questions are directed to the correct person.

Most consultations are conducted in the office, but they can also be virtual or online. If consultations are done online, make sure you are able to contact the surgeon or staff member to ask follow-up questions after you receive your surgical plan. There will always be additional questions, especially when surgery is involved, and particularly when the planned surgery is happening in another state or country.

HOW DID IT GO?

After the consultation, you should fully understand the details of your surgery and aftercare. You may have also made the decision to proceed with your chosen surgeon. However, it is possible that you were left feeling partially informed or unsatisfied with the provider's lackluster and hurried bedside manner. If you have any doubts, it is best to pass on the situation. Keep in mind that the consultation was their opportunity to make a good impression. If their behavior during the consultation is indicative of how they will perform during surgery and post-op, it is likely best to seek another option You deserve the best.

The DC Method™ team is always available to answer questions and provide assistance. Don't hesitate to call if you need information or just someone to listen. Call 866-SCARTLK.

ALWAYS READ BEFORE YOU SIGN

Once you move past the consultation, you will be signing a multitude of disclaimers that essentially prevent you from suing the provider should something go wrong. Signing off on everything is intimidating. Read the documents carefully and ask any additional questions until you have a complete understanding of their policies and the extent of the procedure you are paying for. Once you feel completely at ease, then it's time to sign.

PRO TIP: Take your own before photos of your existing scar or the areas that will be cut during surgery. Take photos from the front and both sides of the area to keep for your personal records."

– Linda Dunn-Carter

While your thorough preparation should help minimize complications should they arise, you'll be happy you kept a detailed record of everything along the way.

CHAPTER 5
AFTERCARE: THE PEARLS AND PITFALLS

The stories I've heard run the gamut. Perhaps you've had surgery and then were disappointed to learn you had no access to critical aftercare. Maybe your doctor never even mentioned how having an aftercare plan could help minimize your risk of scar complications. Or maybe your healing process wasn't exactly "smooth sailing." You might have experienced unexpected complications and unsightly scars that became a depressing after-effect of surgery.

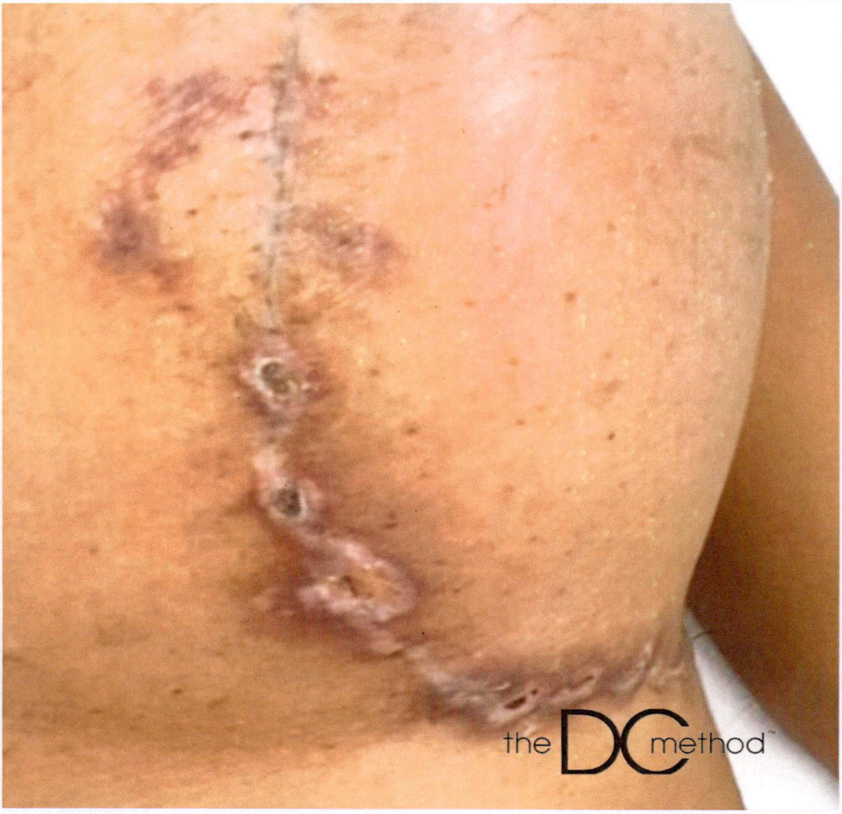

Stream of Spitting Sutures and Erythema

NOWHERE TO TURN

Would you be shocked to learn that many of my patients were unable to contact their doctor directly about post-op issues, much less see them for a follow-up visit? Some patients were relegated to assistants or virtual websites, while others didn't get a callback at all. I can't imagine anything scarier than having to troubleshoot post-op complications on your own. It seems unconscionable, but there it is — the hard truth in many cases.

Having the support of your doctor for aftercare is everything patients hope for - dare I say, what most patients expect. Unfortunately, access to this follow-up care is rarely straightforward. So read on, and we'll share important details on how to forge the path to better aftercare and better healing.

WHAT DRS. DIDN'T TELL THEM. As a scar revision expert, I can't overemphasize the importance of having a post-surgical "Scar Plan." Most doctors won't talk much about the scars that will be left behind after surgery, let alone a Scar Plan. So why do they avoid such basic information? The bare-bones truth is they don't want to scare you out of the surgery. That means it's really up to you to ensure you have a Scar Plan in place. Let that sink in.

It's exciting to have your dream procedure, and maybe all you can think about is how awesome the new you will look!

Maybe you've saved up for Breast Augmentation or a Mommy Makeover and you can't wait to wear a bikini on a tropical island getaway. Not to be a buzzkill, but this is how many of my plastic surgery patients thought before their surgery. With the scars they have now, many wished they never had their surgery in the first place. It's difficult to watch their pain and think that some of the worst complications could have been avoided with pre and post-op planning and proper aftercare.

WHAT MY DOCTOR DIDN'T TELL ME. "My doctors never really discussed aftercare in any detail...." I hear this all too often. Patients report that there might have been a few paragraphs mentioning do's and don'ts in the 50 pages of releases and disclaimers they signed before their surgery. But in their actual meeting pre-op, aftercare is barely discussed, if at all.

Written instructions are typically a standard list of obvious dos and don'ts: Keep the wound clean and dry; use silicone tape; don't do anything to the scar for 6 months; keep the scar protected from the sun; and no lifting or heavy activity for 6 weeks. They might suggest that your scar will fade over the next year or two, but from what I've seen, it's just not reality. For five percent or less of the general surgical population, these tidbits of information might work and voila, your scar isn't that noticeable. However, the other 95% need a whole lot more direction and critical aftercare guidance.

PRO TIP: "The best patient outcomes come from a multidisciplinary approach. While surgery may help some scars, others may be better served by a non-surgical approach. Linda Dunn-Carter uses her scar regimen to break down scars slowly and safely so that they re-heal in a more controlled fashion. She dedicates a lot of time to each patient and each scar to help her patients achieve their goals." *– Dr. Pamela Brownlee, Plastic and Reconstructive Surgeon*

ROUTINE CARE THAT JUST DOESN'T CUT IT

The traditional, old-school aftercare regimen is simply not sufficient. All-in-one scar cream miracles, and silicone tape alone just aren't enough. After witnessing numerous patients with unsuccessful aftercare regimens, I realized the urgency of developing a more effective path to healing and aftercare.

Surveys from my patients continue to testify to this urgent need for good aftercare instructions and at-home products that really work.

> **PRO TIP**: "The vast majority of wounds just don't heal well on their own. Having a Scar Plan that includes in-office procedures and/or Scar Food products is key to a scar's success." – *Linda Dunn-Carter*

WHAT MY DOCTOR DIDN'T TELL ME. Over 90% of my patients admit that their aftercare instructions were lackluster. They were usually left to heal on their own after complications with their incisions. Other times, their healing was challenged by poor suturing that caused open incisions and then infection. They've experienced burns from cannulas that spread over their entire stomachs and spitting sutures that festered under the skin, causing infections, keloids, or hypertrophic scarring. These are nightmare scenarios, and the physical and emotional scars are terrifyingly real.

FINDING AFTERCARE THAT HEALS

The best way to approach aftercare is to educate yourself and understand the phases of healing that your wound will go through. No matter the type of procedure performed, there are many components that impact the scars left on a person's body: the method of wound closure, suturing techniques, the aftercare protocol, and homecare regimens. Let's get started by learning about the major phases of healing that your body will go through.

THE FOUR PHASES OF HEALING

#1*)* **The Hemostasis (clotting) Phase** - This phase includes blood clotting and begins immediately after surgery or injury.

#2) **The Inflammatory Phase - 4-6 days.**
The inflammatory phase includes pain and swelling as controlled bleeding continues from the wound. This inflammation helps to prevent infection, and the natural process of scabbing begins. Inflammation is a natural part of the wound healing process and is only troublesome if it's prolonged or excessive, so you'll want to pass through this phase as quickly as possible. This is also the phase where tape is removed so be extra careful not to accidentally pull sutures out prematurely or re-open your incision.

#3*)* The Proliferative Phase - 4-24 days.
The wound begins to contract and the two edges (margins) of the incision start to merge together. Tension to the incision begins. Healthy looking wounds are pink or red, and by this phase are free from bleeding. The surface can also appear a bit protruding as the edges form together. An unhealthy wound will tend to look dark, and this discoloration can signal infection, inadequate blood flow, or even necrosis (deadening skin).

#4) **The Remodeling (*formation*) Phase - 21 days to 2 years.**
Scar tissue begins to form. Collagen builds, and the wound should be fully closed. Tension to the incision continues. Skin in the wound area will remain weaker for up to 12 weeks. Therefore, extra caution in movement is advised. The length of this phase also depends on various factors, including suture quality, general health and diet, and your post-operative care regime.

ENCOURAGING THE AESTHETIC SCAR

Now that you understand the phases your wound goes through, let's talk about some aftercare techniques that encourage the best aesthetic scar in the end. It all starts with what you do in the beginning to nurture your incision, and doing absolutely nothing is simply not an option! Scars need way more assistance than just silicone tape; they need to be guided and told what to do. Scars need to be *nurtured* back to a healthy state of being, just as if you were nursing yourself back to health from an illness. So, let's get to the good stuff!

The first step of good aftercare is to have all of your products and supplies readily available for use after surgery. **The DC Method**™ takes advantage of recommending our famous aftercare system "Scar Food by **The DC Method**™," which is a range of products with potent ingredients that complement the body's own natural healing process and fast-forwards wound repair.

When can you start Scar Food products?

It's best to start nurturing a new incision with Scar Food products immediately after the surgical tape is removed or when bandages are removed, and of course, after being released from your surgeon's care.

Keep scars hydrated! The old myth of letting scars dry out is long gone and far from proper wound care. Our "Scar Scram Kit" from Scar Food is a complete system that includes a variety of vegan/ organic products specifically designed to apply to a fresh wound or injury. All Scar Food products work synergistically to fast forward the healing process and provide your wound with powerful nutrients.

Scar Food's key nutrients aid in rapid cellular turnover, strengthen new tissue, and help keep the incision moist and pliable to reduce tension. Tension is the culprit in many scar issues, as the skin pulls from both sides of the margin like a tug of war. This kit will be your best friend during the first year of healing.

NEXT

TAPE REMOVAL 3-7 DAYS POST OPERATIVE

Tape removal typically occurs 3-7 days after the operation. Whether you or your surgeon's staff is removing the tape, it must be done slowly to avoid disrupting the incision's integrity. Keep in mind that the skin around the incision site can be very thin, so removing the tape forcefully can potentially damage the skin. I have had patients share horror stories of tape being abruptly ripped off by staff members at their surgeon's office, resulting in not only in tears from the pain but also the incision opening and bleeding. This makes for concerns right at the get go.

So, if you are in the hands of office staff, ask that they tread carefully. If you are removing yourself, I recommend using an oil (like grapeseed or VIT-E oil) and saturating the tape for a minimum of 15 minutes before removal. Once soaked, lift at one end and gently start removing. Keep the tape constantly lubricated with oil as you're removing it inch by inch.

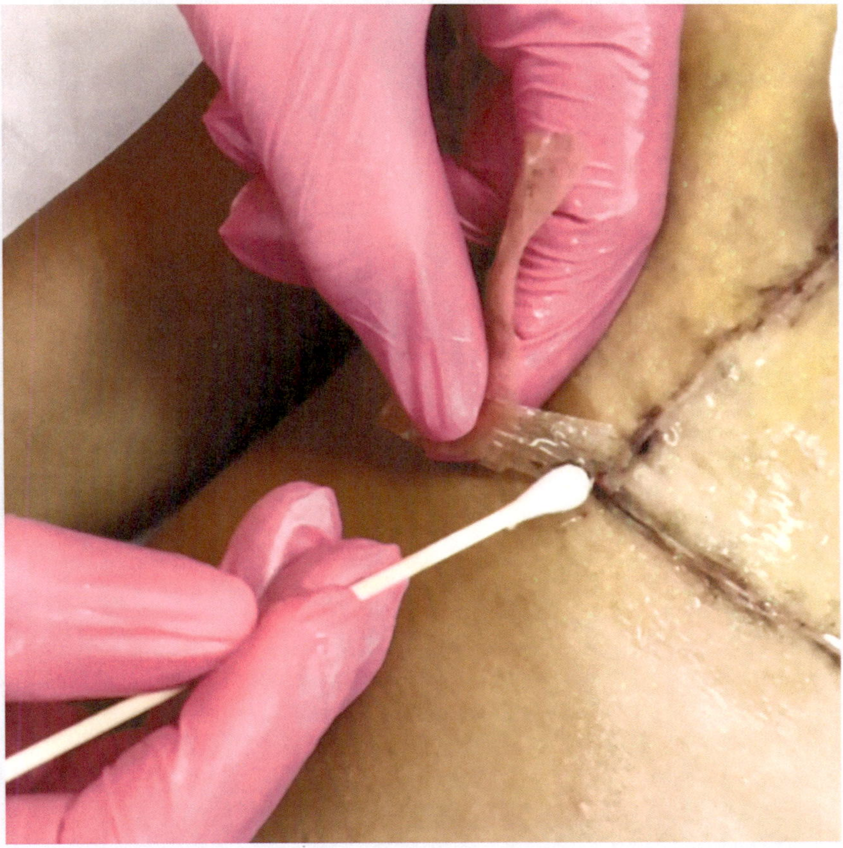

Oil helps to break down the glue on the surgical tape and reduces sensitivity while removing the tape. Pulling the tape off aggressively can cause significant issues, such as opening the incision, pulling out sutures prematurely or tearing the thin skin surrounding the incision.

You should immediately inform your surgeon of any issues, such as **openings of your incision**. If you are unable to see your surgeon right away, over-the-counter butterfly bandages are excellent for temporary use in keeping the incision margins in place. It is also essential to have ointments on hand to prevent infection at the open sites, such as bacitracin, polysporin, or my personal favorite, A&D ointment.

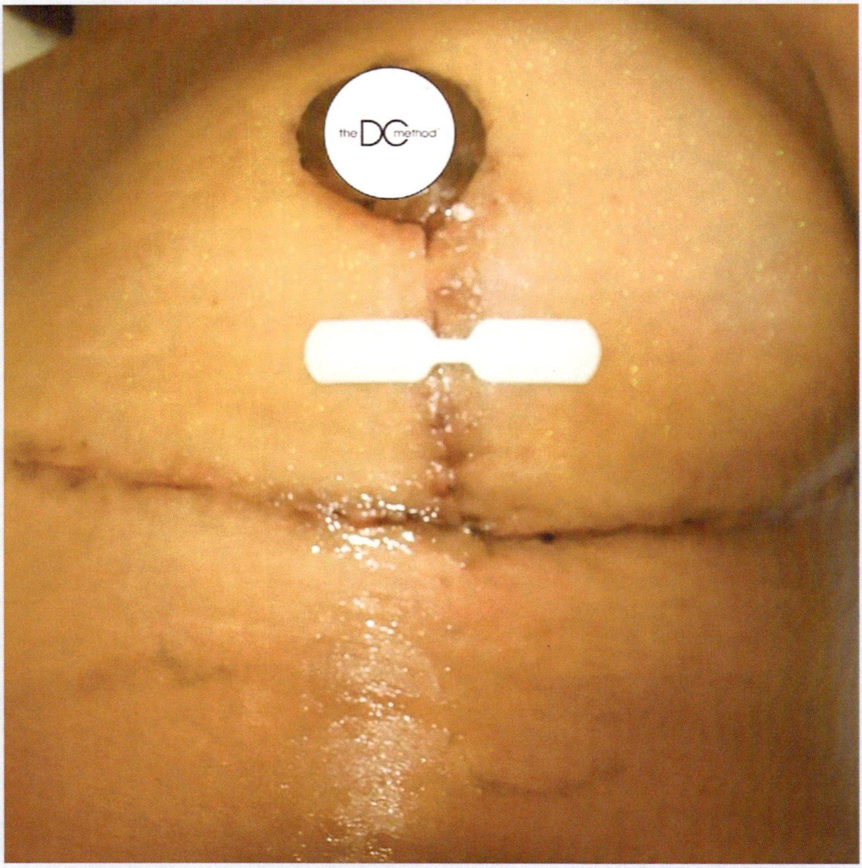

NEXT

Cold Compressions for 2-14 Days

WHY COLD COMPRESSION?

This is a common technique I use after all of my procedures to minimize blood flow after injury and can also be referred to as cryotherapy. You can use cold stones or compresses designed for the freezer or a hot/cold hammer to glide over your incision using the cold side. It really feels soothing on your new incision.

Cold compression is important as it helps to reduce swelling, pain, and inflammation, and it also helps to coagulate blood flow. When used on my patients post-procedure, you can barely tell that their skin was abraded or injured. The less blood flow and inflammation there is in the early stages, the less scarring and potential problems there will be in the end. If you are prone to keloids, this is especially helpful in keeping keloid cells dormant. Keloids can start forming as little as a week after surgery, so cold compression and daily compression wear are extremely beneficial in minimizing blood flow.

Have several Scar Food cold compresses readily available for use immediately after surgery. Apply cold compresses to the wound over your tape and never directly on the skin for 3-5 times a day and 5-15 minutes. Keep compresses in place with an ace bandage or tight clothing.

Cryotherapy chambers can also be great for rapid healing of wounds. Make sure your technician is fully educated on new incisions and how to proceed with therapy with you.

PRO TIP: "Never put cold or hot compresses directly on the skin as it could cause burns. Always use a barrier and don't fall asleep with hot pads on your wounds, as this can also cause burns to the skin." – *Linda Dunn-Carter*

NEXT

COMPRESSION GARMENTS AND WRAPS –

1 day to 6 months depending on the type of surgery, and should be under the direction of your surgeon.

These are absolutely essential to achieve the best outcome for aesthetically appealing scars, **especially** breast lift scars, due to all the weight they bear on the incision. Compression garments and wraps have many benefits, including reducing pain and swelling, minimizing bruising and blood flow, helping to prevent infections, maintaining new body contours, and accelerating the healing process. Compression garments and wraps are **especially** important if you are prone to **keloids** after injury, as they keep blood from flowing to the wound. Blood flow carries cells to the wound that can trigger the start of **keloids**.

NOTE: I see my patients struggling with these suits of armor when they come in for their new scar management series. The strength and muscle twerk it takes to put these garments on, you might as well be in a full-on upper body workout. This is especially concerning if breast lift scars are involved. I'm pretty confident that many of my patients' poor scarring was caused by tension from struggling to pull these suits up and/or snap them together. Just some food for thought, be careful.

SCABBING AFTER INJURY

In principle, it is completely normal for incisions or wounds to have a scab. Your incision might open and bleed, forming a clot (scab).

This is an indication that your incision is healing, but scabs can also cause deeper and wider wound sites. Scabs can form from an open incision, spitting sutures or aftermath of infection. When a scab forms and lies in the seam of your incision or injury, it creates a groove in the skin and becomes vulnerable to premature removal by accidentally rubbing it off with clothing, hitting it on something, or picking at it (for those who pick at scabs).

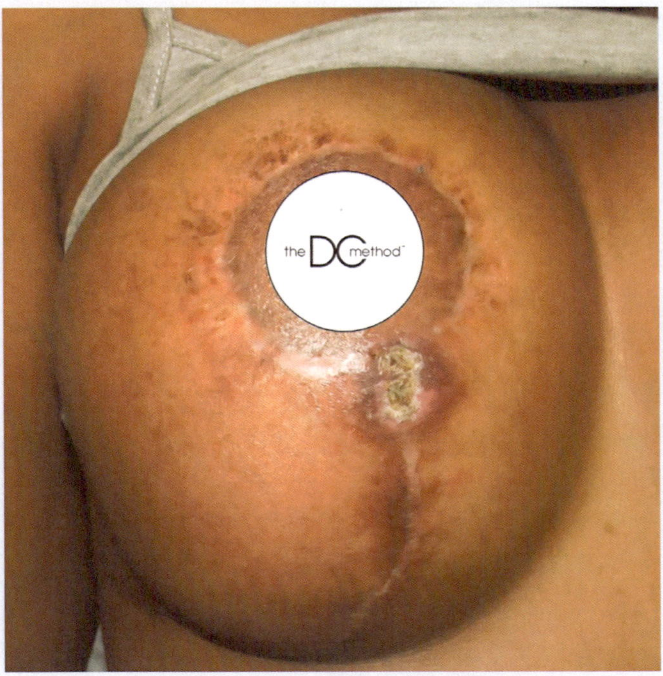

The scab simply gets bigger because it constantly bleeds or oozes from the skin, stretching it. This is not a good situation! It's beneficial to the aesthetic appearance of your scar to bypass scabbing as much as possible by using Scar Food products and protective ointments, such as Bacitracin, Polysporin, or A&D, to help keep scabs moist and encourage faster healing and potentially reduce scarring.

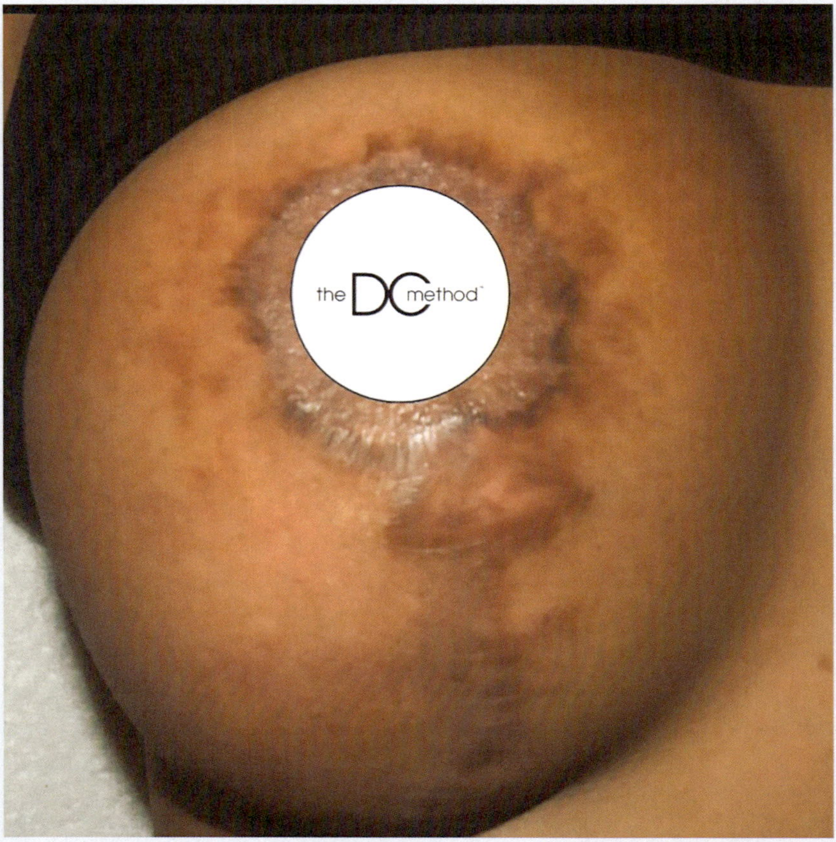

Scab Caused Severe Widening to Scar

MASSAGING - 1 TO 3 MONTHS POST-OP

New wounds, especially sutured wounds, are vulnerable to opening and tension issues, especially in the early phase of healing when the tissue is weak. If you are massaging directly on the skin surrounding the wound, there's a chance you are pulling on that wound and causing more tension along the margins of the incision. The more tension on the incision, the more scarring problems down the road. I realize that lymphatic massages are required after some surgeries, but it's important to make sure your therapist is mindful when stretching the skin around incisions. Even relatively small liposuction incisions can be stretched, causing too much tension and ultimately healing poorly with larger scarring.

Scar tissue begins to form around 3 weeks, and the tissue of your incision starts to strengthen at 2 months. Therefore, if you are massaging, it is important to be extra cautious around those incisions.

IV COCKTAILS - IMMEDIATELY - 1 YEAR

IV drips are very popular to help heal wounds faster. The mixture of certain nutrients can be highly beneficial for scar healing. Drips can also reduce inflammation and promote hydration after surgery. It is crucial to inform your therapist about your current situation so that they can match you with the most suitable cocktail.

NOTE: Make sure to inquire about B & D vitamins used in your drips, as they can contribute to darker melanin, which can darken scars, especially new scars.

HEALTH AND EXERCISE

When it comes to wound healing, it is essential to maintain a healthy lifestyle. Although you cannot work out for many weeks or months, as advised by your surgeon, you can simply walk or use stairs when it is time. Keep moving, but exercise caution as you ease back into your routine. Premature lifting, especially for moms lifting small children, and intense workouts can cause additional tension on the incision and result in more severe scarring. I have observed that scars on the right side of the body tend to be worse, which may be attributed to right-handed individuals, as well as moms who frequently lift their children or engage in household chores. This increased tension and pulling can lead to more severe scarring.

Other important things to avoid are smoking and alcohol.

Alcohol can thin your blood, which makes healing difficult and, in turn, can greatly extend the recovery process. The nicotine and carbon monoxide in cigarettes can interfere with the immune system, delaying healing and increasing the risk of infection at the wound site.

DIET AND MENTAL HEALTH

Maintaining a healthy diet will help your wounds heal faster.

Make an extra effort to include foods with high nutritional value, such as oats, berries, nuts, eggs, and poultry. Other superfoods for healthy healing include yogurt, avocados, chicken broth, turmeric, and vegetables.

Surgery definitely disrupts your normal routine and might even make you a little antsy when homebound, which could lead you to feel a bit depressed. It's important to keep a positive mindset to transfer good vibes to your wound.

Mind over matter can condition your body simply by using your mind to heal. Playing soft meditation music, getting plenty of rest, and speaking positive affirmations to your scar can accelerate recovery and promote positive change.

EXPOSED, SPITTING AND IMPACTED SUTURES

A spitting suture is your body rejecting it and trying to break through the skin. They can be annoying and uncomfortable. You feel like you need to pick or dig for it, which will only make matters worse by disrupting the healthy surrounding tissue and potentially causing more scarring.

It is not uncommon for spitting sutures to appear. Early on, they can look like red pimples or create holes in your skin. If impacted under the skin, they can be painful, start to ooze fluid, become infected, bleed, and then turn into scabs. Spitting sutures can surface immediately after surgery, and I have seen them as late as 8 years post-surgery.

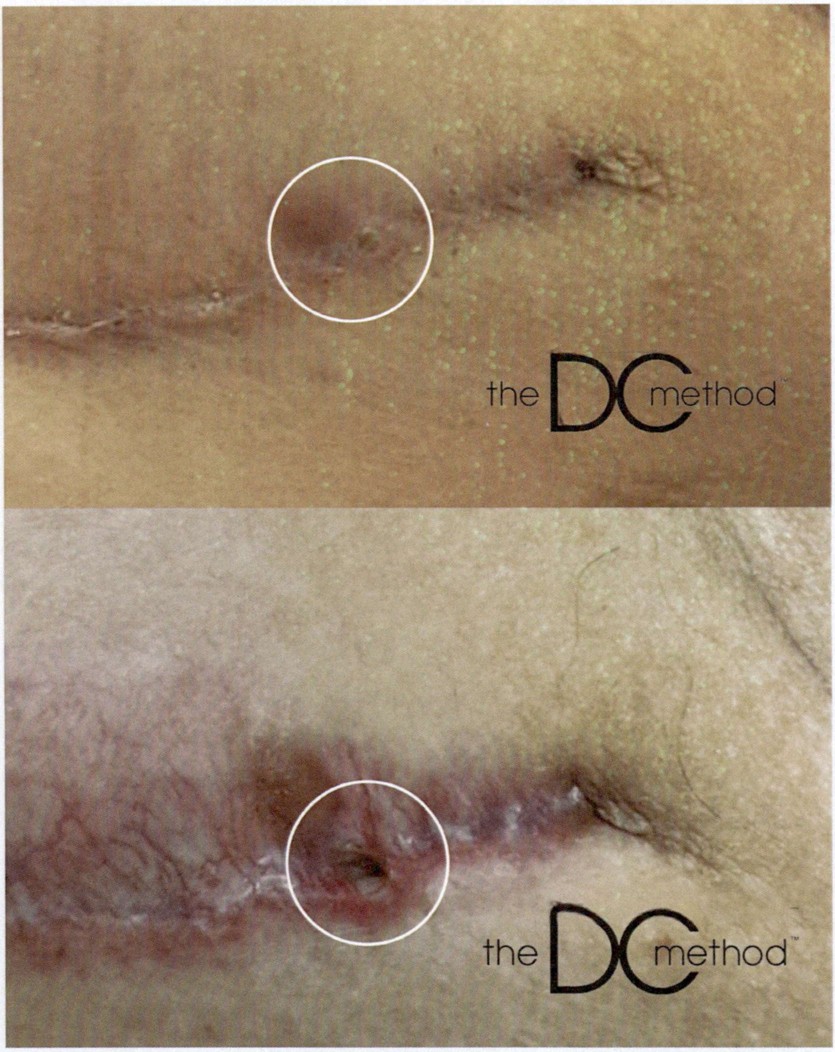

Spitting Suture Under Skin - Top Photo 2 Weeks Post Op, Bottom Photo 3 Weeks. Issues Can Worsen Quickly. Stay Vigilant.

Giving the suture a little tug with sterilized tweezers to see if it will pull out is completely fine. If it doesn't, then simply cut the suture at the skin level; it will most likely dissolve under the skin. Using warm compresses on the impacted areas will also help relieve discomfort. If it's causing more grief than you can manage, it's best to see your doctor or professional practitioner for help.

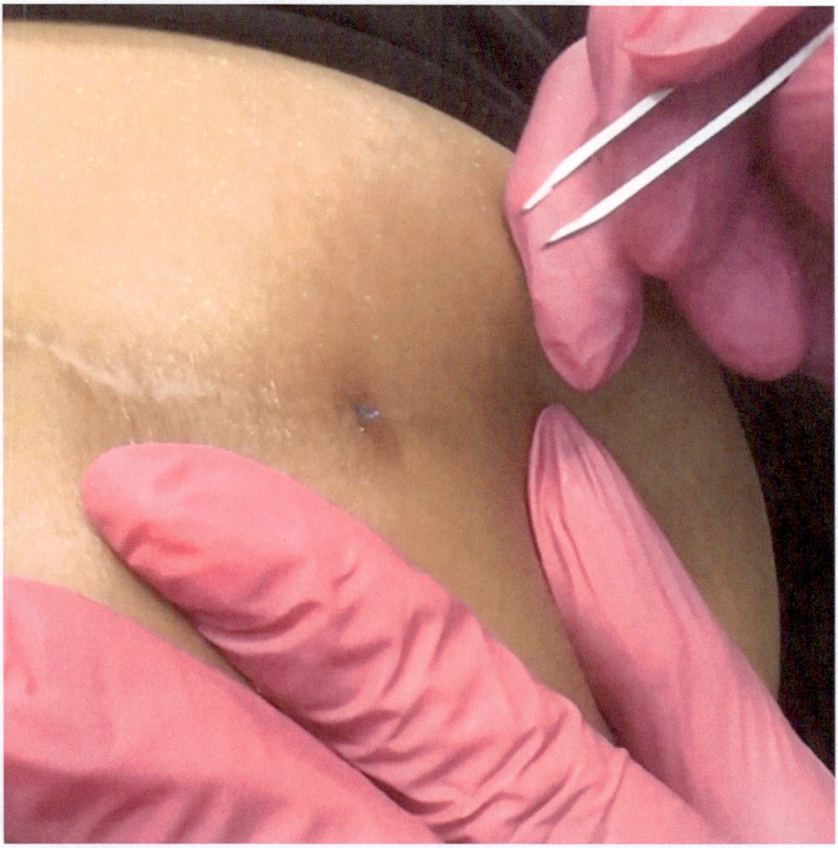

Exposed Spitting Suture

PROTECT YOUR SKIN

A new wound or injury is more delicate than your natural surrounding skin, especially when ultraviolet rays penetrate the clothing and skin. Exposing new tissue to the sun is not advisable as it can cause the area to become red or dark in color. If necessary, adding extra SPF and protective clothing can help prevent damage to delicate scars. After the new incision has healed, it is important to remember that it is still in the formation stage for up to 2 years. This means that the new tissue is more vulnerable to sunburn and sun damage.

A RECAP OF HELPFUL HINTS

- Use Scar Food products to keep the scar area moist immediately out of tape. Wounds that heal in a moist environment are less likely to scar poorly.
- Use cold compresses for up to 10 days when inflammation is at its peak.
- Use compressions: fajas, ace bandages or body wraps. Begin applying them immediately out of tape and continue wearing them for 2-6 months, depending on the type of surgery.
- Limit massages until 1-2 months post-operative, unless lymphatic massage is required.
- Avoid stretching or heavy lifting. Both can cause more stress and tension to the incision, weakening the margins and potentially widening the scar.
- Maintain a healthy diet and a positive mental attitude.
- Use SPF and protective clothing to avoid sun damage to your scars.

SCARS, WHAT DRS. DIDN'T TELL THEM was designed as a resource for all patients considering surgery, or those who have already suffered the devastating impact of scar complications. I hope you have found the book enormously helpful and will continue to use it as a reference guide. My final thoughts are always to do your homework and have a Scar Plan, and I promise you will be on a better path to healing well. The DC Method™ team is here for you anytime you need advice or treatment. Knowledge is power, so never underestimate what it can do for you!

For additional advice and support in scar management, please call 866-SCARTLK or visit my website www.lindadunncarter.com or instagram Lindadunncarter

www.ingramcontent.com/pod-product-compliance
Lightning Source LLC
LaVergne TN
LVRC100954210926
848486LV00018B/402/J

* 9 7 9 8 8 9 2 2 2 2 2 5 9 *